Daily

WELLNESS JOURNAL

-Personal Health Diary and Symptoms Log

DAILY WELLNESS JOURNAL - Personal Health Diary and Symptoms Log

© 2020 B. M. EDITIONS . ALL RIGHTS RESERVED.

ISBN: 9798632947435

CONTENTS

PART ONE

PART TWO

PART THREE

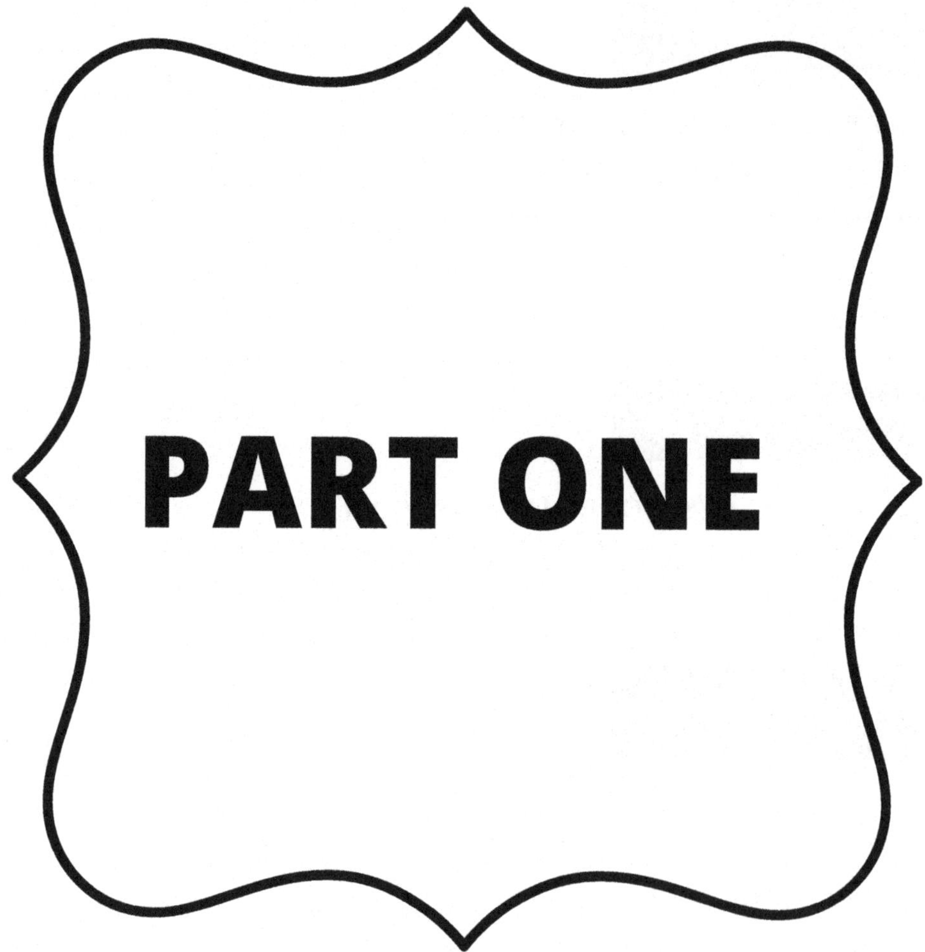

PART ONE

How This Book Can Help You

1. This book can help you if you need a daily, weekly or issue tracker.
2. It is a simple tool, that will allow you to take control of your health and give you peace of mind.
3. It will help you become more aware of yourself and the changes you need to make in your life.
4. This journal helps you not only when you have problems, but also when things are going well.
5. It covers a lot of aspects of your life to help you set goals and have a balanced lifestyle.
6. You can talk to your doctor about this journal and see if there are certain things they would like you to begin recording.
7. It allows you to discuss with your dietician any changes you might make.
8. It contains the information necessary for your annual visit to the doctor.
9. It helps to find the triggers of symptoms and track them.
10. This book can be used to assess pain and fatigue in people with fibromyalgia.
11. You can write about how you are feeling and what kind of pain you are feeling each day.
12. It is a journal that gives good information such as the effect that your diet or the weather can have on your condition.
13. It contains a section for your personal information, medical and surgical history, doctor appointments, medical tests, information for all of your healthcare providers...etc
14. You can also track your screenings, vaccinations, allergies and other information.
15. You can keep track of your activities, the weather and of course how your body is feeling.
16. It will help you know when you took your medication.
17. There is a space where you can write notes/questions that you want to discuss with your doctors.
18. It just takes you 5 minutes to document the whole day.

Personal information

FULL NAME			
DATE OF BIRTH		BIRTH PLACE	
ADDRESS			
CONTACTS			
WEIGHT		HEIGHT	
BLOOD TYPE		EYE COLOR	
EYEGLASSES			
BIRTHMARKS / SCARS			

EMERGENCY CONTACT DETAILS	FULL NAME		RELATIONSHIP	
	ADDRESS		CONTACT NUMBER	

Medical History

PAST SURGICAL PROCEDURES

DATE	PROCEDURE	PHYSICIAN	HOSPITAL

MAJOR ILLNESSES

ILLNESS	START	END	PHYSICIAN	TREATMENT /NOTES

VACCINATIONS

NAME	DATE	NAME	DATE

ALLERGIES

ALLERGY	REACTION	ALLERGY	REACTION

Family History

MOTHER'S SIDE

NAME	RELATIONSHIP	CONDITION /ILLNESS	AGE OF ONSET	CAUSE OF DEATH	AGE AT DEATH

FATHER'S SIDE

NAME	RELATIONSHIP	CONDITION /ILLNESS	AGE OF ONSET	CAUSE OF DEATH	AGE AT DEATH

SIBLINGS

NAME	RELATIONSHIP	CONDITION /ILLNESS	AGE OF ONSET	CAUSE OF DEATH	AGE AT DEATH

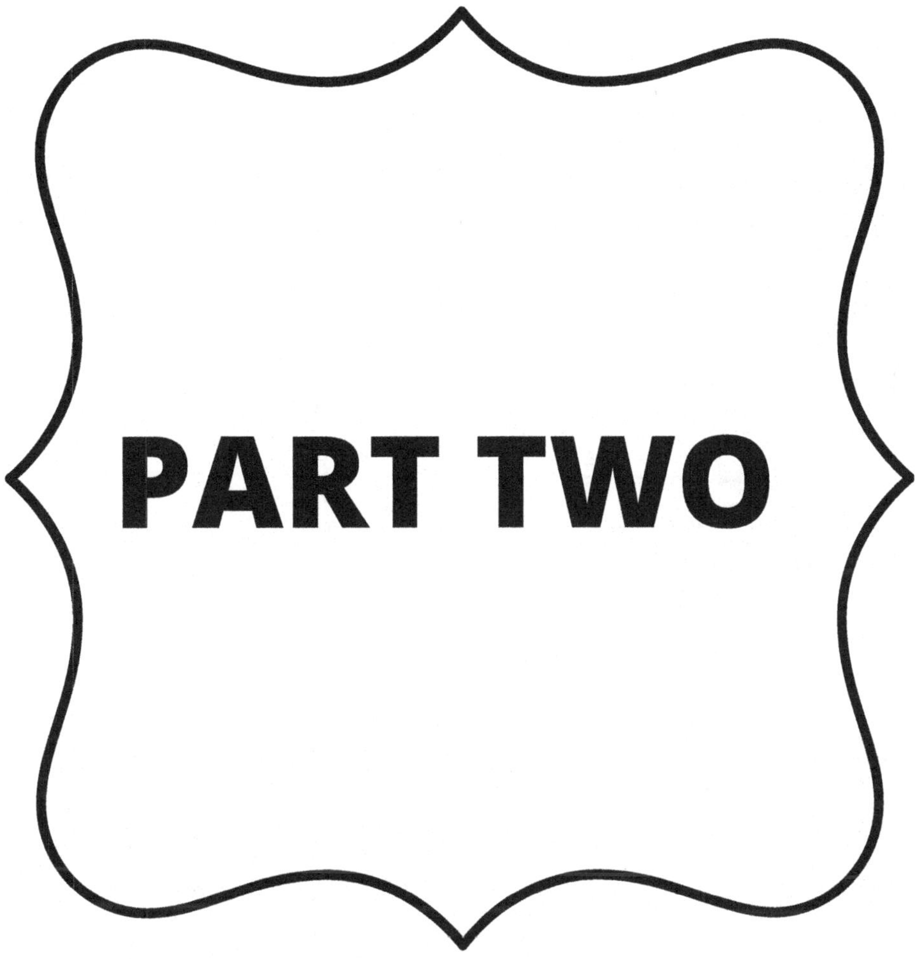

PART TWO

DATE: 6.19 DAY: Monday

DAILY QUOTE

"Nothing too small in our life for the [illegible] answers all prayers."

	AM	PM
WEIGHT	129	
TEMPERATURE		
BLOOD PRESSURE		

SUGAR LEVEL

BEFORE BREAKFAST :	AFTER BREAKFAST:
BEFORE LUNCH :	AFTER LUNCH :
BEFORE DINNER :	AFTER DINNER :

BEDTIME :

SLEEP LAST NIGHT

6 ½ /HOURS

☐ ☺ ☒ ☹ ☐ 😫

NAPS TODAY

☐ /TOTAL HOURS ☐ /HOW MANY

DRUGS/VITAMINS /HERBS/MEDICATIONS	REASON	DOSAGE	TIME			REACTION
VITAMIN B1	JOINTS	250mg	8	0	0	✓
VITAMIN B12	BRAIN FOG	250mg	"	"	"	✓

SYMPTOM NOTES

RECURRING SYMPTOMS	headache
NEW SYMPTOMS	

PAIN SITE IDENTIFICATION

x4

MARK PAINFUL AREAS OF THE BODY

OVERALL MORNING PAIN LEVEL

(1) 2 3 4 5 6 7 8 9 10

LOW HIGH

OVERALL AFTERNOON PAIN LEVEL

1 2 (3) 4 5 6 7 8 9 10

LOW HIGH

OVERALL EVENING PAIN LEVEL

1 2 3 4 5 6 7 8 9 10

LOW HIGH

SUSPECTED TRIGGERS

Always Sugar

MEDICATIONS: NA

DID THE MEDICATION HELP? NA

PHYSICAL ACTIVITY

ACTIVITY/ EXERCISE	DURATION	SETS	REPS	CAL	NOTES
Work	3hrs				

FATIGUE

1 2 3 4 5 6 7 8 9 10

DEPRESSION / ANXIETY

1 (2) 3 4 5 6 7 8 9 10

MOOD

☆☆☆☆☆

TODAY'S DIET

WATER INTAKE
lemon water

BREAKFAST TIME : 7:00
1 Coffee
1 Egg 8:30
CAL : .... CARBS: .... PROTEIN .... FAT ....

LUNCH TIME : ....
CAL : .... CARBS: .... PROTEIN .... FAT ....

DINNER TIME : ....
CAL : .... CARBS: .... PROTEIN .... FAT ....

SNACKS TIME: ....
CAL : .... CARBS: .... PROTEIN .... FAT ....

REACTION TO FOODS

MEAL : ....
FOOD : ....

SYMPTOMS

....

HOW MY APPETITE AFFECTED ?
1 2 3 4 5 6 7 8 9 10
NOT AFFECTED NO APPETITE

HOW IS MY URINATION
1 2 3 4 5 6 7 8 9 10
GOOD WORST

HOW IS MY BOWELS
1 2 3 4 5 6 7 8 9 10
CONSTIPATED LOOSE

EXACERBATING CONDITIONS

CURENT WEATHER
SUNNY OVERCAST (circled)
FOGGY
RAINY SNOWY

CURRENT WEATHER AFFECTING ME
1 2 3 4 5 6 7 8 9 10
NONE GREATLY

JOB STRESS LEVEL
1 2 3 (circled) 4 5 6 7 8 9 10
LOW HIGH

TEMPERATURE
LOW HIGH

FAMILY HOME LIFE STRESS LEVEL
1 (circled) 2 3 4 5 6 7 8 9 10
LOW HIGH

TOP 3 THINGS I WILL DO TO MY CARE-SELF TODAY
EAT WELL

TOP 3 THINGS TO ACCOMPLISH TODAY
COOK
GARDEN

TOP 3 HIGHLIGHTS OF MY DAY

NOTES /COMMENTS

River

DATE: 6·26 DAY:

Sam-E

DAILY QUOTE

	AM	PM
WEIGHT	129	
TEMPERATURE		
BLOOD PRESSURE		

SUGAR LEVEL

BEFORE BREAKFAST :	AFTER BREAKFAST:
BEFORE LUNCH :	AFTER LUNCH :
BEFORE DINNER :	AFTER DINNER :

BEDTIME :

SLEEP LAST NIGHT

/HOURS

NAPS TODAY

/TOTAL HOURS /HOW MANY

DRUGS/VITAMINS /HERBS/MEDICATIONS	REASON	DOSAGE	TIME			REACTION

SYMPTOM NOTES

RECURRING SYMPTOMS	TOXIC ??
NEW SYMPTOMS	↑headache MAGNESIUM 400 mg / day POTASSIUM 500mg to 2000 Methyl FOLATE

PAIN SITE IDENTIFICATION

MARK PAINFUL AREAS OF THE BODY

OVERALL MORNING PAIN LEVEL

1 2 3 4 5 6 7 8 9 10

LOW HIGH

OVERALL AFTERNOON PAIN LEVEL

1 2 3 4 5 6 7 8 9 10

LOW HIGH

OVERALL EVENING PAIN LEVEL

1 2 3 4 5 6 7 8 9 10

LOW HIGH

SUSPECTED TRIGGERS

MEDICATIONS:

DID THE MEDICATION HELP?

PHYSICAL ACTIVITY

ACTIVITY/ EXERCISE	DURATION	SETS	REPS	CAL	NOTES

FATIGUE

1 2 3 4 5 6 7 8 9 10

DEPRESSION / ANXIETY

1 2 3 4 5 6 7 8 9 10

MOOD

☆☆☆☆☆

TODAY'S DIET

WATER INTAKE

BREAKFAST TIME : ....

....
....
....
....

CAL : .... CARBS: .... PROTEIN .... FAT ....

LUNCH TIME : ....

....
....
....
....

CAL : .... CARBS: .... PROTEIN .... FAT ....

DINNER TIME : ....

....
....
....
....

CAL : .... CARBS: .... PROTEIN .... FAT ....

SNACKS TIME: ....

....
....
....
....

CAL : .... CARBS: .... PROTEIN .... FAT ....

REACTION TO FOODS

MEAL : ....

FOOD : ....

SYMPTOMS

....
....
....
....
....

HOW MY APPETITE AFFECTED ?

1 2 3 4 5 6 7 8 9 10

NOT AFFECTED NO APPETITE

HOW IS MY URINATION

1 2 3 4 5 6 7 8 9 10

GOOD WORST

HOW IS MY BOWELS

1 2 3 4 5 6 7 8 9 10

CONSTIPATED LOOSE

EXACERBATING CONDITIONS

CURENT WEATHER

SUNNY OVERCAST

FOGGY

RAINY SNOWY

CURRENT WEATHER AFFECTING ME

1 2 3 4 5 6 7 8 9 10

NONE GREATLY

JOB STRESS LEVEL

1 2 3 4 5 6 7 8 9 10

LOW HIGH

TEMPERATURE

LOW HIGH

FAMILY HOME LIFE STRESS LEVEL

1 2 3 4 5 6 7 8 9 10

LOW HIGH

TOP 3 THINGS I WILL DO TO MY CARE-SELF TODAY

....
....
....

TOP 3 THINGS TO ACCOMPLISH TODAY

....
....
....

TOP 3 HIGHLIGHTS OF MY DAY

....
....
....

NOTES /COMMENTS

....
....
....
....

DATE: .... DAY: ....

DAILY QUOTE

"..
...."

	AM	PM
WEIGHT		
TEMPERATURE		
BLOOD PRESSURE		

SUGAR LEVEL

BEFORE BREAKFAST :	AFTER BREAKFAST:
BEFORE LUNCH :	AFTER LUNCH :
BEFORE DINNER :	AFTER DINNER :

BEDTIME :

SLEEP LAST NIGHT

☐ /HOURS

☐ ☺ ☐ ☹ ☐

NAPS TODAY

☐ /TOTAL HOURS ☐ /HOW MANY

DRUGS/VITAMINS /HERBS/MEDICATIONS	REASON	DOSAGE	TIME			REACTION

SYMPTOM NOTES

RECURRING SYMPTOMS	
NEW SYMPTOMS	

PAIN SITE IDENTIFICATION

MARK PAINFUL AREAS OF THE BODY

OVERALL MORNING PAIN LEVEL

1 2 3 4 5 6 7 8 9 10

LOW HIGH

OVERALL EVENING PAIN LEVEL

1 2 3 4 5 6 7 8 9 10

LOW HIGH

OVERALL AFTERNOON PAIN LEVEL

1 2 3 4 5 6 7 8 9 10

LOW HIGH

SUSPECTED TRIGGERS

....
....

MEDICATIONS: ....

DID THE MEDICATION HELP? ....

PHYSICAL ACTIVITY

ACTIVITY/ EXERCISE	DURATION	SETS	REPS	CAL	NOTES

FATIGUE

1 2 3 4 5 6 7 8 9 10

DEPRESSION / ANXIETY

1 2 3 4 5 6 7 8 9 10

MOOD

☆☆☆☆☆

TODAY'S DIET

WATER INTAKE

BREAKFAST TIME : ....

...

CAL : .... CARBS: .... PROTEIN .... FAT ....

LUNCH TIME : ....

...

CAL : .... CARBS: .... PROTEIN .... FAT ....

DINNER TIME : ....

...

CAL : .... CARBS: .... PROTEIN .... FAT ....

SNACKS TIME: ....

...

CAL : .... CARBS: .... PROTEIN .... FAT ....

REACTION TO FOODS

MEAL : ....

FOOD : ....

SYMPTOMS

...

HOW MY APPETITE AFFECTED ?

1 2 3 4 5 6 7 8 9 10

NOT AFFECTED NO APPETITE

HOW IS MY URINATION

1 2 3 4 5 6 7 8 9 10

GOOD WORST

HOW IS MY BOWELS

1 2 3 4 5 6 7 8 9 10

CONSTIPATED LOOSE

EXACERBATING CONDITIONS

CURENT WEATHER

SUNNY OVERCAST

FOGGY

RAINY SNOWY

CURRENT WEATHER AFFECTING ME

1 2 3 4 5 6 7 8 9 10

NONE GREATLY

JOB STRESS LEVEL

1 2 3 4 5 6 7 8 9 10

LOW HIGH

TEMPERATURE

LOW HIGH

FAMILY HOME LIFE STRESS LEVEL

1 2 3 4 5 6 7 8 9 10

LOW HIGH

TOP 3 THINGS I WILL DO TO MY CARE-SELF TODAY

...

TOP 3 THINGS TO ACCOMPLISH TODAY

...

TOP 3 HIGHLIGHTS OF MY DAY

...

NOTES /COMMENTS

...

DATE: .... DAY: ....

DAILY QUOTE

"..
...."

	AM	PM
WEIGHT		
TEMPERATURE		
BLOOD PRESSURE		

SUGAR LEVEL

BEFORE BREAKFAST :	AFTER BREAKFAST:
BEFORE LUNCH :	AFTER LUNCH :
BEFORE DINNER :	AFTER DINNER :

BEDTIME :

SLEEP LAST NIGHT

☐ /HOURS

☐ ☺ ☐ ☹ ☐

NAPS TODAY

☐ /TOTAL HOURS ☐ /HOW MANY

DRUGS/VITAMINS /HERBS/MEDICATIONS	REASON	DOSAGE	TIME			REACTION

SYMPTOM NOTES

RECURRING SYMPTOMS	
NEW SYMPTOMS	

PAIN SITE IDENTIFICATION

MARK PAINFUL AREAS OF THE BODY

OVERALL MORNING PAIN LEVEL

1 2 3 4 5 6 7 8 9 10

LOW HIGH

OVERALL AFTERNOON PAIN LEVEL

1 2 3 4 5 6 7 8 9 10

LOW HIGH

OVERALL EVENING PAIN LEVEL

1 2 3 4 5 6 7 8 9 10

LOW HIGH

SUSPECTED TRIGGERS

....
....

MEDICATIONS: ....

DID THE MEDICATION HELP? ....

PHYSICAL ACTIVITY

ACTIVITY/ EXERCISE	DURATION	SETS	REPS	CAL	NOTES

FATIGUE

1 2 3 4 5 6 7 8 9 10

DEPRESSION / ANXIETY

1 2 3 4 5 6 7 8 9 10

MOOD

☆☆☆☆☆

TODAY'S DIET

WATER INTAKE

BREAKFAST TIME : ....

....

....

....

....

CAL : .... CARBS: .... PROTEIN .... FAT ....

LUNCH TIME : ....

....

....

....

....

CAL : .... CARBS: .... PROTEIN .... FAT ....

DINNER TIME : ....

....

....

....

....

CAL : .... CARBS: .... PROTEIN .... FAT ....

SNACKS TIME: ....

....

....

....

....

CAL : .... CARBS: .... PROTEIN .... FAT ....

REACTION TO FOODS

MEAL : ....

FOOD : ....

SYMPTOMS

....

....

....

....

....

HOW MY APPETITE AFFECTED ?

1 2 3 4 5 6 7 8 9 10

NOT AFFECTED NO APPETITE

HOW IS MY URINATION

1 2 3 4 5 6 7 8 9 10

GOOD WORST

HOW IS MY BOWELS

1 2 3 4 5 6 7 8 9 10

CONSTIPATED LOOSE

EXACERBATING CONDITIONS

CURENT WEATHER

SUNNY OVERCAST

FOGGY

RAINY SNOWY

CURRENT WEATHER AFFECTING ME

1 2 3 4 5 6 7 8 9 10

NONE GREATLY

JOB STRESS LEVEL

1 2 3 4 5 6 7 8 9 10

LOW HIGH

TEMPERATURE

LOW HIGH

FAMILY HOME LIFE STRESS LEVEL

1 2 3 4 5 6 7 8 9 10

LOW HIGH

TOP 3 THINGS I WILL DO TO MY CARE-SELF TODAY

....

....

....

TOP 3 THINGS TO ACCOMPLISH TODAY

....

....

....

TOP 3 HIGHLIGHTS OF MY DAY

....

....

....

NOTES /COMMENTS

....

....

....

....

DATE: .... DAY: ....

DAILY QUOTE

" ....
.... "

	AM	PM
WEIGHT		
TEMPERATURE		
BLOOD PRESSURE		

SUGAR LEVEL

BEFORE BREAKFAST :	AFTER BREAKFAST:
BEFORE LUNCH :	AFTER LUNCH :
BEFORE DINNER :	AFTER DINNER :

BEDTIME :

SLEEP LAST NIGHT

☐ /HOURS

☐ ☺ ☐ ☹ ☐

NAPS TODAY

☐ /TOTAL HOURS ☐ /HOW MANY

DRUGS/VITAMINS /HERBS/MEDICATIONS	REASON	DOSAGE	TIME			REACTION

SYMPTOM NOTES

RECURRING SYMPTOMS	
NEW SYMPTOMS	

PAIN SITE IDENTIFICATION

MARK PAINFUL AREAS OF THE BODY

OVERALL MORNING PAIN LEVEL

1 2 3 4 5 6 7 8 9 10

LOW HIGH

OVERALL AFTERNOON PAIN LEVEL

1 2 3 4 5 6 7 8 9 10

LOW HIGH

OVERALL EVENING PAIN LEVEL

1 2 3 4 5 6 7 8 9 10

LOW HIGH

SUSPECTED TRIGGERS

....
....

MEDICATIONS: ....

DID THE MEDICATION HELP? ....

PHYSICAL ACTIVITY

ACTIVITY/ EXERCISE	DURATION	SETS	REPS	CAL	NOTES

FATIGUE

1 2 3 4 5 6 7 8 9 10

DEPRESSION / ANXIETY

1 2 3 4 5 6 7 8 9 10

MOOD

☆ ☆ ☆ ☆ ☆

TODAY'S DIET

WATER INTAKE

BREAKFAST TIME : ....

....
....
....
....

CAL : .... CARBS: .... PROTEIN .... FAT ....

LUNCH TIME : ....

....
....
....
....

CAL : .... CARBS: .... PROTEIN .... FAT ....

DINNER TIME : ....

....
....
....
....

CAL : .... CARBS: .... PROTEIN .... FAT ....

SNACKS TIME: ....

....
....
....
....

CAL : .... CARBS: .... PROTEIN .... FAT ....

REACTION TO FOODS

MEAL : ....

FOOD : ....

SYMPTOMS

....
....
....
....
....

HOW MY APPETITE AFFECTED ?

1 2 3 4 5 6 7 8 9 10

NOT AFFECTED NO APPETITE

HOW IS MY URINATION

1 2 3 4 5 6 7 8 9 10

GOOD WORST

HOW IS MY BOWELS

1 2 3 4 5 6 7 8 9 10

CONSTIPATED LOOSE

EXACERBATING CONDITIONS

CURENT WEATHER

SUNNY OVERCAST

FOGGY

RAINY SNOWY

CURRENT WEATHER AFFECTING ME

1 2 3 4 5 6 7 8 9 10

NONE GREATLY

JOB STRESS LEVEL

1 2 3 4 5 6 7 8 9 10

LOW HIGH

TEMPERATURE

LOW HIGH

FAMILY HOME LIFE STRESS LEVEL

1 2 3 4 5 6 7 8 9 10

LOW HIGH

TOP 3 THINGS I WILL DO TO MY CARE-SELF TODAY

....
....
....

TOP 3 THINGS TO ACCOMPLISH TODAY

....
....
....

TOP 3 HIGHLIGHTS OF MY DAY

....
....
....

NOTES /COMMENTS

....
....
....
....

DATE: .... DAY: ....

DAILY QUOTE

"
....
....
"

	AM	PM
WEIGHT		
TEMPERATURE		
BLOOD PRESSURE		

SUGAR LEVEL

BEFORE BREAKFAST :	AFTER BREAKFAST:
BEFORE LUNCH :	AFTER LUNCH :
BEFORE DINNER :	AFTER DINNER :
BEDTIME :	

SLEEP LAST NIGHT

☐ /HOURS

☐ ☺ ☐ ☹ ☐

NAPS TODAY

☐ /TOTAL HOURS ☐ /HOW MANY

DRUGS/VITAMINS /HERBS/MEDICATIONS	REASON	DOSAGE	TIME			REACTION

SYMPTOM NOTES

RECURRING SYMPTOMS	
NEW SYMPTOMS	

PAIN SITE IDENTIFICATION

MARK PAINFUL AREAS OF THE BODY

OVERALL MORNING PAIN LEVEL

1 2 3 4 5 6 7 8 9 10

LOW HIGH

OVERALL EVENING PAIN LEVEL

1 2 3 4 5 6 7 8 9 10

LOW HIGH

OVERALL AFTERNOON PAIN LEVEL

1 2 3 4 5 6 7 8 9 10

LOW HIGH

SUSPECTED TRIGGERS

....
....

MEDICATIONS: ....

DID THE MEDICATION HELP? ....

PHYSICAL ACTIVITY

ACTIVITY/ EXERCISE	DURATION	SETS	REPS	CAL	NOTES

FATIGUE

1 2 3 4 5 6 7 8 9 10

DEPRESSION / ANXIETY

1 2 3 4 5 6 7 8 9 10

MOOD

☆ ☆ ☆ ☆ ☆

TODAY'S DIET

WATER INTAKE

BREAKFAST TIME :

CAL : CARBS: PROTEIN FAT

LUNCH TIME :

CAL : CARBS: PROTEIN FAT

DINNER TIME :

CAL : CARBS: PROTEIN FAT

SNACKS TIME:

CAL : CARBS: PROTEIN FAT

REACTION TO FOODS

MEAL :

FOOD :

SYMPTOMS

HOW MY APPETITE AFFECTED ?

1 2 3 4 5 6 7 8 9 10

NOT AFFECTED NO APPETITE

HOW IS MY URINATION

1 2 3 4 5 6 7 8 9 10

GOOD WORST

HOW IS MY BOWELS

1 2 3 4 5 6 7 8 9 10

CONSTIPATED LOOSE

EXACERBATING CONDITIONS

CURENT WEATHER

SUNNY OVERCAST

FOGGY

RAINY SNOWY

CURRENT WEATHER AFFECTING ME

1 2 3 4 5 6 7 8 9 10

NONE GREATLY

TEMPERATURE

LOW HIGH

JOB STRESS LEVEL

1 2 3 4 5 6 7 8 9 10

LOW HIGH

FAMILY HOME LIFE STRESS LEVEL

1 2 3 4 5 6 7 8 9 10

LOW HIGH

TOP 3 THINGS I WILL DO TO MY CARE-SELF TODAY

TOP 3 THINGS TO ACCOMPLISH TODAY

TOP 3 HIGHLIGHTS OF MY DAY

NOTES /COMMENTS

DATE: .... DAY: ....

DAILY QUOTE

"..
...."

	AM	PM
WEIGHT		
TEMPERATURE		
BLOOD PRESSURE		

SUGAR LEVEL

BEFORE BREAKFAST :	AFTER BREAKFAST:
BEFORE LUNCH :	AFTER LUNCH :
BEFORE DINNER :	AFTER DINNER :

BEDTIME :

SLEEP LAST NIGHT

☐ /HOURS

☐ ☺ ☐ ☹ ☐

NAPS TODAY

☐ /TOTAL HOURS ☐ /HOW MANY

DRUGS/VITAMINS /HERBS/MEDICATIONS	REASON	DOSAGE	TIME			REACTION

SYMPTOM NOTES

RECURRING SYMPTOMS	
NEW SYMPTOMS	

PAIN SITE IDENTIFICATION

MARK PAINFUL AREAS OF THE BODY

OVERALL MORNING PAIN LEVEL

1 2 3 4 5 6 7 8 9 10

LOW HIGH

OVERALL AFTERNOON PAIN LEVEL

1 2 3 4 5 6 7 8 9 10

LOW HIGH

OVERALL EVENING PAIN LEVEL

1 2 3 4 5 6 7 8 9 10

LOW HIGH

SUSPECTED TRIGGERS

....
....

MEDICATIONS: ....

DID THE MEDICATION HELP? ....

PHYSICAL ACTIVITY

ACTIVITY/ EXERCISE	DURATION	SETS	REPS	CAL	NOTES

FATIGUE

1 2 3 4 5 6 7 8 9 10

DEPRESSION / ANXIETY

1 2 3 4 5 6 7 8 9 10

MOOD

☆ ☆ ☆ ☆ ☆

TODAY'S DIET

WATTER INTAKE

BREAKFAST TIME : ....

....

CAL : .... CARBS: .... PROTEIN .... FAT ....

LUNCH TIME : ....

....

CAL : .... CARBS: .... PROTEIN .... FAT ....

DINNER TIME : ....

....

CAL : .... CARBS: .... PROTEIN .... FAT ....

SNACKS TIME: ....

....

CAL : .... CARBS: .... PROTEIN .... FAT ....

REACTION TO FOODS

MEAL : ....

FOOD : ....

SYMPTOMS

....

HOW MY APPETITE AFFECTED ?

1 2 3 4 5 6 7 8 9 10

NOT AFFECTED NO APPETITE

HOW IS MY URINATION

1 2 3 4 5 6 7 8 9 10

GOOD WORST

HOW IS MY BOWELS

1 2 3 4 5 6 7 8 9 10

CONSTIPATED LOOSE

EXACERBATING CONDITIONS

CURENT WEATHER

SUNNY OVERCAST

FOGGY

RAINY SNOWY

CURRENT WEATHER AFFECTING ME

1 2 3 4 5 6 7 8 9 10

NONE GREATLY

JOB STRESS LEVEL

1 2 3 4 5 6 7 8 9 10

LOW HIGH

TEMPERATURE

LOW HIGH

FAMILY HOME LIFE STRESS LEVEL

1 2 3 4 5 6 7 8 9 10

LOW HIGH

TOP 3 THINGS I WILL DO TO MY CARE-SELF TODAY

....

TOP 3 THINGS TO ACCOMPLISH TODAY

....

TOP 3 HIGHLIGHTS OF MY DAY

....

NOTES /COMMENTS

....

DATE: .... DAY: ....

DAILY QUOTE

"..
...."

	AM	PM
WEIGHT		
TEMPERATURE		
BLOOD PRESSURE		

SUGAR LEVEL

BEFORE BREAKFAST :	AFTER BREAKFAST:
BEFORE LUNCH :	AFTER LUNCH :
BEFORE DINNER :	AFTER DINNER :

BEDTIME :

SLEEP LAST NIGHT

☐ /HOURS

☐ ☺ ☐ ☹ ☐ 😫

NAPS TODAY

☐ /TOTAL HOURS ☐ /HOW MANY

DRUGS/VITAMINS /HERBS/MEDICATIONS	REASON	DOSAGE	TIME			REACTION

SYMPTOM NOTES

RECURRING SYMPTOMS	
NEW SYMPTOMS	

PAIN SITE IDENTIFICATION

MARK PAINFUL AREAS OF THE BODY

OVERALL MORNING PAIN LEVEL

1 2 3 4 5 6 7 8 9 10

LOW HIGH

OVERALL EVENING PAIN LEVEL

1 2 3 4 5 6 7 8 9 10

LOW HIGH

OVERALL AFTERNOON PAIN LEVEL

1 2 3 4 5 6 7 8 9 10

LOW HIGH

SUSPECTED TRIGGERS

....
....

MEDICATIONS: ....

DID THE MEDICATION HELP? ....

PHYSICAL ACTIVITY

ACTIVITY/ EXERCISE	DURATION	SETS	REPS	CAL	NOTES

FATIGUE

1 2 3 4 5 6 7 8 9 10

DEPRESSION / ANXIETY

1 2 3 4 5 6 7 8 9 10

MOOD

☆☆☆☆☆

TODAY'S DIET

WATER INTAKE

BREAKFAST TIME : ....

....

....

....

....

CAL : .... CARBS: .... PROTEIN .... FAT ....

LUNCH TIME : ....

....

....

....

....

CAL : .... CARBS: .... PROTEIN .... FAT ....

DINNER TIME : ....

....

....

....

....

CAL : .... CARBS: .... PROTEIN .... FAT ....

SNACKS TIME: ....

....

....

....

....

CAL : .... CARBS: .... PROTEIN .... FAT ....

REACTION TO FOODS

MEAL : ....

FOOD : ....

SYMPTOMS

....

....

....

....

....

HOW MY APPETITE AFFECTED ?

1 2 3 4 5 6 7 8 9 10

NOT AFFECTED NO APPETITE

HOW IS MY URINATION

1 2 3 4 5 6 7 8 9 10

GOOD WORST

HOW IS MY BOWELS

1 2 3 4 5 6 7 8 9 10

CONSTIPATED LOOSE

EXACERBATING CONDITIONS

CURENT WEATHER

SUNNY OVERCAST

FOGGY

RAINY SNOWY

CURRENT WEATHER AFFECTING ME

1 2 3 4 5 6 7 8 9 10

NONE GREATLY

JOB STRESS LEVEL

1 2 3 4 5 6 7 8 9 10

LOW HIGH

TEMPERATURE

LOW HIGH

FAMILY HOME LIFE STRESS LEVEL

1 2 3 4 5 6 7 8 9 10

LOW HIGH

TOP 3 THINGS I WILL DO TO MY CARE-SELF TODAY

....

....

....

TOP 3 THINGS TO ACCOMPLISH TODAY

....

....

....

TOP 3 HIGHLIGHTS OF MY DAY

....

....

....

NOTES /COMMENTS

....

....

....

....

DATE: .... DAY: ....

DAILY QUOTE

" ....
.... "

	AM	PM
WEIGHT		
TEMPERATURE		
BLOOD PRESSURE		

SUGAR LEVEL

BEFORE BREAKFAST :	AFTER BREAKFAST:
BEFORE LUNCH :	AFTER LUNCH :
BEFORE DINNER :	AFTER DINNER :

BEDTIME :

SLEEP LAST NIGHT

☐ /HOURS

☐ ☺ ☐ ☹ ☐

NAPS TODAY

☐ /TOTAL HOURS ☐ /HOW MANY

DRUGS/VITAMINS /HERBS/MEDICATIONS	REASON	DOSAGE	TIME			REACTION

SYMPTOM NOTES

RECURRING SYMPTOMS	
NEW SYMPTOMS	

PAIN SITE IDENTIFICATION

MARK PAINFUL AREAS OF THE BODY

OVERALL MORNING PAIN LEVEL

1 2 3 4 5 6 7 8 9 10

LOW HIGH

OVERALL AFTERNOON PAIN LEVEL

1 2 3 4 5 6 7 8 9 10

LOW HIGH

OVERALL EVENING PAIN LEVEL

1 2 3 4 5 6 7 8 9 10

LOW HIGH

SUSPECTED TRIGGERS

....
....

MEDICATIONS: ....

DID THE MEDICATION HELP? ....

PHYSICAL ACTIVITY

ACTIVITY/ EXERCISE	DURATION	SETS	REPS	CAL	NOTES

FATIGUE

1 2 3 4 5 6 7 8 9 10

DEPRESSION / ANXIETY

1 2 3 4 5 6 7 8 9 10

MOOD

☆☆☆☆☆

TODAY'S DIET

WATER INTAKE

BREAKFAST TIME : ....

....
....
....
....

CAL : .... CARBS: .... PROTEIN .... FAT ....

LUNCH TIME : ....

....
....
....
....

CAL : .... CARBS: .... PROTEIN .... FAT ....

DINNER TIME : ....

....
....
....
....

CAL : .... CARBS: .... PROTEIN .... FAT ....

SNACKS TIME: ....

....
....
....
....

CAL : .... CARBS: .... PROTEIN .... FAT ....

REACTION TO FOODS

MEAL : ....

FOOD : ....

SYMPTOMS

....
....
....
....
....

HOW MY APPETITE AFFECTED ?

1 2 3 4 5 6 7 8 9 10

NOT AFFECTED NO APPETITE

HOW IS MY URINATION

1 2 3 4 5 6 7 8 9 10

GOOD WORST

HOW IS MY BOWELS

1 2 3 4 5 6 7 8 9 10

CONSTIPATED LOOSE

EXACERBATING CONDITIONS

CURENT WEATHER

SUNNY OVERCAST

FOGGY

RAINY SNOWY

CURRENT WEATHER AFFECTING ME

1 2 3 4 5 6 7 8 9 10

NONE GREATLY

JOB STRESS LEVEL

1 2 3 4 5 6 7 8 9 10

LOW HIGH

TEMPERATURE

LOW HIGH

FAMILY HOME LIFE STRESS LEVEL

1 2 3 4 5 6 7 8 9 10

LOW HIGH

TOP 3 THINGS I WILL DO TO MY CARE-SELF TODAY

....
....
....

TOP 3 THINGS TO ACCOMPLISH TODAY

....
....
....

TOP 3 HIGHLIGHTS OF MY DAY

....
....
....

NOTES /COMMENTS

....
....
....
....

DATE: .... **DAY:** ....

DAILY QUOTE

" ....
.... "

	AM	PM
WEIGHT		
TEMPERATURE		
BLOOD PRESSURE		

SUGAR LEVEL

BEFORE BREAKFAST :	AFTER BREAKFAST:
BEFORE LUNCH :	AFTER LUNCH :
BEFORE DINNER :	AFTER DINNER :
BEDTIME :	

SLEEP LAST NIGHT

☐ /HOURS

☐ ☺ ☐ ☹ ☐ 😫

NAPS TODAY

☐ /TOTAL HOURS ☐ /HOW MANY

DRUGS/VITAMINS /HERBS/MEDICATIONS	REASON	DOSAGE	TIME			REACTION

SYMPTOM NOTES

RECURRING SYMPTOMS	
NEW SYMPTOMS	

PAIN SITE IDENTIFICATION

MARK PAINFUL AREAS OF THE BODY

OVERALL MORNING PAIN LEVEL

1 2 3 4 5 6 7 8 9 10

LOW HIGH

OVERALL AFTERNOON PAIN LEVEL

1 2 3 4 5 6 7 8 9 10

LOW HIGH

OVERALL EVENING PAIN LEVEL

1 2 3 4 5 6 7 8 9 10

LOW HIGH

SUSPECTED TRIGGERS

....
....

MEDICATIONS: ....

DID THE MEDICATION HELP? ....

PHYSICAL ACTIVITY

ACTIVITY/ EXERCISE	DURATION	SETS	REPS	CAL	NOTES

FATIGUE

1 2 3 4 5 6 7 8 9 10

DEPRESSION / ANXIETY

1 2 3 4 5 6 7 8 9 10

MOOD

☆☆☆☆☆

TODAY'S DIET

WATER INTAKE

BREAKFAST TIME :

CAL : CARBS: PROTEIN FAT

LUNCH TIME :

CAL : CARBS: PROTEIN FAT

DINNER TIME :

CAL : CARBS: PROTEIN FAT

SNACKS TIME:

CAL : CARBS: PROTEIN FAT

REACTION TO FOODS

MEAL :

FOOD :

SYMPTOMS

HOW MY APPETITE AFFECTED ?

1 2 3 4 5 6 7 8 9 10

NOT AFFECTED NO APPETITE

HOW IS MY URINATION

1 2 3 4 5 6 7 8 9 10

GOOD WORST

HOW IS MY BOWELS

1 2 3 4 5 6 7 8 9 10

CONSTIPATED LOOSE

EXACERBATING CONDITIONS

CURENT WEATHER

SUNNY OVERCAST

FOGGY

RAINY SNOWY

CURRENT WEATHER AFFECTING ME

1 2 3 4 5 6 7 8 9 10

NONE GREATLY

JOB STRESS LEVEL

1 2 3 4 5 6 7 8 9 10

LOW HIGH

TEMPERATURE

LOW HIGH

FAMILY HOME LIFE STRESS LEVEL

1 2 3 4 5 6 7 8 9 10

LOW HIGH

TOP 3 THINGS I WILL DO TO MY CARE-SELF TODAY

TOP 3 THINGS TO ACCOMPLISH TODAY

TOP 3 HIGHLIGHTS OF MY DAY

NOTES /COMMENTS

DATE: .... DAY: ....

DAILY QUOTE

"
....
.... "

	AM	PM
WEIGHT		
TEMPERATURE		
BLOOD PRESSURE		

SUGAR LEVEL

BEFORE BREAKFAST :	AFTER BREAKFAST:
BEFORE LUNCH :	AFTER LUNCH :
BEFORE DINNER :	AFTER DINNER :

BEDTIME :

SLEEP LAST NIGHT

☐ /HOURS

☐ ☺ ☐ ☹ ☐

NAPS TODAY

☐ /TOTAL HOURS ☐ /HOW MANY

DRUGS/VITAMINS /HERBS/MEDICATIONS	REASON	DOSAGE	TIME			REACTION

SYMPTOM NOTES

RECURRING SYMPTOMS	
NEW SYMPTOMS	

PAIN SITE IDENTIFICATION

MARK PAINFUL AREAS OF THE BODY

OVERALL MORNING PAIN LEVEL

1 2 3 4 5 6 7 8 9 10

LOW HIGH

OVERALL AFTERNOON PAIN LEVEL

1 2 3 4 5 6 7 8 9 10

LOW HIGH

OVERALL EVENING PAIN LEVEL

1 2 3 4 5 6 7 8 9 10

LOW HIGH

SUSPECTED TRIGGERS

....
....

MEDICATIONS: ....

DID THE MEDICATION HELP? ....

PHYSICAL ACTIVITY

ACTIVITY/ EXERCISE	DURATION	SETS	REPS	CAL	NOTES

FATIGUE

1 2 3 4 5 6 7 8 9 10

DEPRESSION / ANXIETY

1 2 3 4 5 6 7 8 9 10

MOOD

☆☆☆☆☆

TODAY'S DIET

WATER INTAKE

BREAKFAST TIME : ....

....

CAL : .... CARBS: .... PROTEIN .... FAT ....

LUNCH TIME : ....

....

CAL : .... CARBS: .... PROTEIN .... FAT ....

DINNER TIME : ....

....

CAL : .... CARBS: .... PROTEIN .... FAT ....

SNACKS TIME: ....

....

CAL : .... CARBS: .... PROTEIN .... FAT ....

REACTION TO FOODS

MEAL : ....

FOOD : ....

SYMPTOMS

....

HOW MY APPETITE AFFECTED ?

1 2 3 4 5 6 7 8 9 10

NOT AFFECTED NO APPETITE

HOW IS MY URINATION

1 2 3 4 5 6 7 8 9 10

GOOD WORST

HOW IS MY BOWELS

1 2 3 4 5 6 7 8 9 10

CONSTIPATED LOOSE

EXACERBATING CONDITIONS

CURENT WEATHER

SUNNY OVERCAST

FOGGY

RAINY SNOWY

CURRENT WEATHER AFFECTING ME

1 2 3 4 5 6 7 8 9 10

NONE GREATLY

JOB STRESS LEVEL

1 2 3 4 5 6 7 8 9 10

LOW HIGH

TEMPERATURE

LOW HIGH

FAMILY HOME LIFE STRESS LEVEL

1 2 3 4 5 6 7 8 9 10

LOW HIGH

TOP 3 THINGS I WILL DO TO MY CARE-SELF TODAY

....

TOP 3 THINGS TO ACCOMPLISH TODAY

....

TOP 3 HIGHLIGHTS OF MY DAY

....

NOTES /COMMENTS

....

DATE: .... DAY: ....

DAILY QUOTE

"..
...."

	AM	PM
WEIGHT		
TEMPERATURE		
BLOOD PRESSURE		

SUGAR LEVEL

BEFORE BREAKFAST :	AFTER BREAKFAST:
BEFORE LUNCH :	AFTER LUNCH :
BEFORE DINNER :	AFTER DINNER :

BEDTIME :

SLEEP LAST NIGHT

☐ /HOURS

☐ ☺ ☐ ☹ ☐

NAPS TODAY

☐ /TOTAL HOURS ☐ /HOW MANY

DRUGS/VITAMINS /HERBS/MEDICATIONS	REASON	DOSAGE	TIME			REACTION

SYMPTOM NOTES

RECURRING SYMPTOMS	
NEW SYMPTOMS	

PAIN SITE IDENTIFICATION

MARK PAINFUL AREAS OF THE BODY

OVERALL MORNING PAIN LEVEL

1 2 3 4 5 6 7 8 9 10

LOW HIGH

OVERALL AFTERNOON PAIN LEVEL

1 2 3 4 5 6 7 8 9 10

LOW HIGH

OVERALL EVENING PAIN LEVEL

1 2 3 4 5 6 7 8 9 10

LOW HIGH

SUSPECTED TRIGGERS

....
....

MEDICATIONS: ....

DID THE MEDICATION HELP? ....

PHYSICAL ACTIVITY

ACTIVITY/ EXERCISE	DURATION	SETS	REPS	CAL	NOTES

FATIGUE

1 2 3 4 5 6 7 8 9 10

DEPRESSION / ANXIETY

1 2 3 4 5 6 7 8 9 10

MOOD

☆☆☆☆☆

TODAY'S DIET

WATER INTAKE

BREAKFAST TIME : ....

CAL : .... CARBS: .... PROTEIN .... FAT ....

LUNCH TIME : ....

CAL : .... CARBS: .... PROTEIN .... FAT ....

DINNER TIME : ....

CAL : .... CARBS: .... PROTEIN .... FAT ....

SNACKS TIME: ....

CAL : .... CARBS: .... PROTEIN .... FAT ....

REACTION TO FOODS

MEAL : ....

FOOD : ....

SYMPTOMS

HOW MY APPETITE AFFECTED ?

1 2 3 4 5 6 7 8 9 10

NOT AFFECTED NO APPETITE

HOW IS MY URINATION

1 2 3 4 5 6 7 8 9 10

GOOD WORST

HOW IS MY BOWELS

1 2 3 4 5 6 7 8 9 10

CONSTIPATED LOOSE

EXACERBATING CONDITIONS

CURENT WEATHER

SUNNY OVERCAST

FOGGY

RAINY SNOWY

CURRENT WEATHER AFFECTING ME

1 2 3 4 5 6 7 8 9 10

NONE GREATLY

JOB STRESS LEVEL

1 2 3 4 5 6 7 8 9 10

LOW HIGH

TEMPERATURE

LOW HIGH

FAMILY HOME LIFE STRESS LEVEL

1 2 3 4 5 6 7 8 9 10

LOW HIGH

TOP 3 THINGS I WILL DO TO MY CARE-SELF TODAY

TOP 3 THINGS TO ACCOMPLISH TODAY

TOP 3 HIGHLIGHTS OF MY DAY

NOTES /COMMENTS

DATE: .... DAY: ....

DAILY QUOTE

"..
...."

	AM	PM
WEIGHT		
TEMPERATURE		
BLOOD PRESSURE		

SUGAR LEVEL

BEFORE BREAKFAST :	AFTER BREAKFAST:
BEFORE LUNCH :	AFTER LUNCH :
BEFORE DINNER :	AFTER DINNER :
BEDTIME :	

SLEEP LAST NIGHT

☐ /HOURS

☐ ☐ ☐

NAPS TODAY

☐ /TOTAL HOURS ☐ /HOW MANY

DRUGS/VITAMINS /HERBS/MEDICATIONS	REASON	DOSAGE	TIME			REACTION

SYMPTOM NOTES

RECURRING SYMPTOMS	
NEW SYMPTOMS	

PAIN SITE IDENTIFICATION

MARK PAINFUL AREAS OF THE BODY

OVERALL MORNING PAIN LEVEL
1 2 3 4 5 6 7 8 9 10
LOW HIGH

OVERALL AFTERNOON PAIN LEVEL
1 2 3 4 5 6 7 8 9 10
LOW HIGH

OVERALL EVENING PAIN LEVEL
1 2 3 4 5 6 7 8 9 10
LOW HIGH

SUSPECTED TRIGGERS

....
....

MEDICATIONS: ....

DID THE MEDICATION HELP? ....

PHYSICAL ACTIVITY

ACTIVITY/ EXERCISE	DURATION	SETS	REPS	CAL	NOTES

FATIGUE
1 2 3 4 5 6 7 8 9 10

DEPRESSION / ANXIETY
1 2 3 4 5 6 7 8 9 10

MOOD
☆☆☆☆☆

TODAY'S DIET

WATER INTAKE

BREAKFAST TIME : ....

....

....

....

....

CAL : .... CARBS: .... PROTEIN .... FAT ....

LUNCH TIME : ....

....

....

....

....

CAL : .... CARBS: .... PROTEIN .... FAT ....

DINNER TIME : ....

....

....

....

....

CAL : .... CARBS: .... PROTEIN .... FAT ....

SNACKS TIME: ....

....

....

....

....

CAL : .... CARBS: .... PROTEIN .... FAT ....

REACTION TO FOODS

MEAL : ....

FOOD : ....

SYMPTOMS

....

....

....

....

....

HOW MY APPETITE AFFECTED ?

1 2 3 4 5 6 7 8 9 10

NOT AFFECTED NO APPETITE

HOW IS MY URINATION

1 2 3 4 5 6 7 8 9 10

GOOD WORST

HOW IS MY BOWELS

1 2 3 4 5 6 7 8 9 10

CONSTIPATED LOOSE

EXACERBATING CONDITIONS

CURENT WEATHER

SUNNY OVERCAST

FOGGY

RAINY SNOWY

CURRENT WEATHER AFFECTING ME

1 2 3 4 5 6 7 8 9 10

NONE GREATLY

JOB STRESS LEVEL

1 2 3 4 5 6 7 8 9 10

LOW HIGH

TEMPERATURE

LOW HIGH

FAMILY HOME LIFE STRESS LEVEL

1 2 3 4 5 6 7 8 9 10

LOW HIGH

TOP 3 THINGS I WILL DO TO MY CARE-SELF TODAY

....

....

....

TOP 3 THINGS TO ACCOMPLISH TODAY

....

....

....

TOP 3 HIGHLIGHTS OF MY DAY

....

....

....

NOTES /COMMENTS

....

....

....

....

DATE: .... DAY: ....

DAILY QUOTE

"..
...."

	AM	PM
WEIGHT		
TEMPERATURE		
BLOOD PRESSURE		

SUGAR LEVEL

BEFORE BREAKFAST :	AFTER BREAKFAST:
BEFORE LUNCH :	AFTER LUNCH :
BEFORE DINNER :	AFTER DINNER :

BEDTIME :

SLEEP LAST NIGHT

☐ /HOURS

☐ ☺ ☐ ☹ ☐

NAPS TODAY

☐ /TOTAL HOURS ☐ /HOW MANY

DRUGS/VITAMINS /HERBS/MEDICATIONS	REASON	DOSAGE	TIME			REACTION

SYMPTOM NOTES

RECURRING SYMPTOMS	
NEW SYMPTOMS	

PAIN SITE IDENTIFICATION

MARK PAINFUL AREAS OF THE BODY

OVERALL MORNING PAIN LEVEL

1 2 3 4 5 6 7 8 9 10

LOW HIGH

OVERALL AFTERNOON PAIN LEVEL

1 2 3 4 5 6 7 8 9 10

LOW HIGH

OVERALL EVENING PAIN LEVEL

1 2 3 4 5 6 7 8 9 10

LOW HIGH

SUSPECTED TRIGGERS

....
....

MEDICATIONS: ....

DID THE MEDICATION HELP? ....

PHYSICAL ACTIVITY

ACTIVITY/ EXERCISE	DURATION	SETS	REPS	CAL	NOTES

FATIGUE

1 2 3 4 5 6 7 8 9 10

DEPRESSION / ANXIETY

1 2 3 4 5 6 7 8 9 10

MOOD

☆☆☆☆☆

TODAY'S DIET

WATER INTAKE

BREAKFAST TIME : ....

CAL : .... CARBS: .... PROTEIN .... FAT ....

LUNCH TIME : ....

CAL : .... CARBS: .... PROTEIN .... FAT ....

DINNER TIME : ....

CAL : .... CARBS: .... PROTEIN .... FAT ....

SNACKS TIME: ....

CAL : .... CARBS: .... PROTEIN .... FAT ....

REACTION TO FOODS

MEAL : ....

FOOD : ....

SYMPTOMS

HOW MY APPETITE AFFECTED ?

1 2 3 4 5 6 7 8 9 10

NOT AFFECTED NO APPETITE

HOW IS MY URINATION

1 2 3 4 5 6 7 8 9 10

GOOD WORST

HOW IS MY BOWELS

1 2 3 4 5 6 7 8 9 10

CONSTIPATED LOOSE

EXACERBATING CONDITIONS

CURENT WEATHER

SUNNY OVERCAST

FOGGY

RAINY SNOWY

CURRENT WEATHER AFFECTING ME

1 2 3 4 5 6 7 8 9 10

NONE GREATLY

JOB STRESS LEVEL

1 2 3 4 5 6 7 8 9 10

LOW HIGH

TEMPERATURE

LOW HIGH

FAMILY HOME LIFE STRESS LEVEL

1 2 3 4 5 6 7 8 9 10

LOW HIGH

TOP 3 THINGS I WILL DO TO MY CARE-SELF TODAY

TOP 3 THINGS TO ACCOMPLISH TODAY

TOP 3 HIGHLIGHTS OF MY DAY

NOTES /COMMENTS

DATE: .... DAY: ....

DAILY QUOTE

" ....
.... "

	AM	PM
WEIGHT		
TEMPERATURE		
BLOOD PRESSURE		

SUGAR LEVEL

BEFORE BREAKFAST :	AFTER BREAKFAST:
BEFORE LUNCH :	AFTER LUNCH :
BEFORE DINNER :	AFTER DINNER :

BEDTIME :

SLEEP LAST NIGHT

☐ /HOURS

☐ ☐ ☐

NAPS TODAY

☐ /TOTAL HOURS ☐ /HOW MANY

DRUGS/VITAMINS /HERBS/MEDICATIONS	REASON	DOSAGE	TIME			REACTION

SYMPTOM NOTES

RECURRING SYMPTOMS	
NEW SYMPTOMS	

PAIN SITE IDENTIFICATION

MARK PAINFUL AREAS OF THE BODY

OVERALL MORNING PAIN LEVEL

1 2 3 4 5 6 7 8 9 10

LOW HIGH

OVERALL AFTERNOON PAIN LEVEL

1 2 3 4 5 6 7 8 9 10

LOW HIGH

OVERALL EVENING PAIN LEVEL

1 2 3 4 5 6 7 8 9 10

LOW HIGH

SUSPECTED TRIGGERS

....
....

MEDICATIONS: ....

DID THE MEDICATION HELP? ....

PHYSICAL ACTIVITY

ACTIVITY/ EXERCISE	DURATION	SETS	REPS	CAL	NOTES

FATIGUE

1 2 3 4 5 6 7 8 9 10

DEPRESSION / ANXIETY

1 2 3 4 5 6 7 8 9 10

MOOD

☆☆☆☆☆

TODAY'S DIET

WATER INTAKE

BREAKFAST TIME : ....

CAL : .... CARBS: .... PROTEIN .... FAT ....

LUNCH TIME : ....

CAL : .... CARBS: .... PROTEIN .... FAT ....

DINNER TIME : ....

CAL : .... CARBS: .... PROTEIN .... FAT ....

SNACKS TIME: ....

CAL : .... CARBS: .... PROTEIN .... FAT ....

REACTION TO FOODS

MEAL : ....

FOOD : ....

SYMPTOMS

HOW MY APPETITE AFFECTED ?

1 2 3 4 5 6 7 8 9 10

NOT AFFECTED NO APPETITE

HOW IS MY URINATION

1 2 3 4 5 6 7 8 9 10

GOOD WORST

HOW IS MY BOWELS

1 2 3 4 5 6 7 8 9 10

CONSTIPATED LOOSE

EXACERBATING CONDITIONS

CURENT WEATHER

SUNNY OVERCAST

FOGGY

RAINY SNOWY

CURRENT WEATHER AFFECTING ME

1 2 3 4 5 6 7 8 9 10

NONE GREATLY

JOB STRESS LEVEL

1 2 3 4 5 6 7 8 9 10

LOW HIGH

TEMPERATURE

LOW HIGH

FAMILY HOME LIFE STRESS LEVEL

1 2 3 4 5 6 7 8 9 10

LOW HIGH

TOP 3 THINGS I WILL DO TO MY CARE-SELF TODAY

TOP 3 THINGS TO ACCOMPLISH TODAY

TOP 3 HIGHLIGHTS OF MY DAY

NOTES /COMMENTS

DATE: .... DAY: ....

DAILY QUOTE

"..
...."

	AM	PM
WEIGHT		
TEMPERATURE		
BLOOD PRESSURE		

SUGAR LEVEL

BEFORE BREAKFAST :	AFTER BREAKFAST:
BEFORE LUNCH :	AFTER LUNCH :
BEFORE DINNER :	AFTER DINNER :
BEDTIME :	

SLEEP LAST NIGHT

☐ /HOURS

☐ ☺ ☐ ☹ ☐

NAPS TODAY

☐ /TOTAL HOURS ☐ /HOW MANY

DRUGS/VITAMINS /HERBS/MEDICATIONS	REASON	DOSAGE	TIME			REACTION

SYMPTOM NOTES

RECURRING SYMPTOMS	
NEW SYMPTOMS	

PAIN SITE IDENTIFICATION

MARK PAINFUL AREAS OF THE BODY

OVERALL MORNING PAIN LEVEL

1 2 3 4 5 6 7 8 9 10

LOW HIGH

OVERALL AFTERNOON PAIN LEVEL

1 2 3 4 5 6 7 8 9 10

LOW HIGH

OVERALL EVENING PAIN LEVEL

1 2 3 4 5 6 7 8 9 10

LOW HIGH

SUSPECTED TRIGGERS

....
....

MEDICATIONS: ....

DID THE MEDICATION HELP? ....

PHYSICAL ACTIVITY

ACTIVITY/ EXERCISE	DURATION	SETS	REPS	CAL	NOTES

FATIGUE

1 2 3 4 5 6 7 8 9 10

DEPRESSION / ANXIETY

1 2 3 4 5 6 7 8 9 10

MOOD

☆☆☆☆☆

TODAY'S DIET

WATER INTAKE

BREAKFAST TIME : ....

....

....

....

....

CAL : .... CARBS: .... PROTEIN .... FAT ....

LUNCH TIME : ....

....

....

....

....

CAL : .... CARBS: .... PROTEIN .... FAT ....

DINNER TIME : ....

....

....

....

....

CAL : .... CARBS: .... PROTEIN .... FAT ....

SNACKS TIME: ....

....

....

....

....

CAL : .... CARBS: .... PROTEIN .... FAT ....

REACTION TO FOODS

MEAL : ....

FOOD : ....

SYMPTOMS

....

....

....

....

....

HOW MY APPETITE AFFECTED ?

1 2 3 4 5 6 7 8 9 10

NOT AFFECTED NO APPETITE

HOW IS MY URINATION

1 2 3 4 5 6 7 8 9 10

GOOD WORST

HOW IS MY BOWELS

1 2 3 4 5 6 7 8 9 10

CONSTIPATED LOOSE

EXACERBATING CONDITIONS

CURENT WEATHER

SUNNY OVERCAST

FOGGY

RAINY SNOWY

CURRENT WEATHER AFFECTING ME

1 2 3 4 5 6 7 8 9 10

NONE GREATLY

JOB STRESS LEVEL

1 2 3 4 5 6 7 8 9 10

LOW HIGH

TEMPERATURE

LOW HIGH

FAMILY HOME LIFE STRESS LEVEL

1 2 3 4 5 6 7 8 9 10

LOW HIGH

TOP 3 THINGS I WILL DO TO MY CARE-SELF TODAY

....

....

....

TOP 3 THINGS TO ACCOMPLISH TODAY

....

....

....

TOP 3 HIGHLIGHTS OF MY DAY

....

....

....

NOTES /COMMENTS

....

....

....

....

DATE: .... DAY: ....

DAILY QUOTE

"..
...."

	AM	PM
WEIGHT		
TEMPERATURE		
BLOOD PRESSURE		

SUGAR LEVEL

BEFORE BREAKFAST :	AFTER BREAKFAST:
BEFORE LUNCH :	AFTER LUNCH :
BEFORE DINNER :	AFTER DINNER :
BEDTIME :	

SLEEP LAST NIGHT

/HOURS

NAPS TODAY

/TOTAL HOURS /HOW MANY

DRUGS/VITAMINS /HERBS/MEDICATIONS	REASON	DOSAGE	TIME			REACTION

SYMPTOM NOTES

RECURRING SYMPTOMS	
NEW SYMPTOMS	

PAIN SITE IDENTIFICATION

MARK PAINFUL AREAS OF THE BODY

OVERALL MORNING PAIN LEVEL

1 2 3 4 5 6 7 8 9 10

LOW HIGH

OVERALL EVENING PAIN LEVEL

1 2 3 4 5 6 7 8 9 10

LOW HIGH

OVERALL AFTERNOON PAIN LEVEL

1 2 3 4 5 6 7 8 9 10

LOW HIGH

SUSPECTED TRIGGERS

....
....

MEDICATIONS: ....

DID THE MEDICATION HELP? ....

PHYSICAL ACTIVITY

ACTIVITY/ EXERCISE	DURATION	SETS	REPS	CAL	NOTES

FATIGUE

1 2 3 4 5 6 7 8 9 10

DEPRESSION / ANXIETY

1 2 3 4 5 6 7 8 9 10

MOOD

☆☆☆☆☆

TODAY'S DIET

WATER INTAKE

BREAKFAST TIME : ....

CAL : .... CARBS: .... PROTEIN .... FAT ....

LUNCH TIME : ....

CAL : .... CARBS: .... PROTEIN .... FAT ....

DINNER TIME : ....

CAL : .... CARBS: .... PROTEIN .... FAT ....

SNACKS TIME: ....

CAL : .... CARBS: .... PROTEIN .... FAT ....

REACTION TO FOODS

MEAL : ....

FOOD : ....

SYMPTOMS

HOW MY APPETITE AFFECTED ?

1 2 3 4 5 6 7 8 9 10

NOT AFFECTED NO APPETITE

HOW IS MY URINATION

1 2 3 4 5 6 7 8 9 10

GOOD WORST

HOW IS MY BOWELS

1 2 3 4 5 6 7 8 9 10

CONSTIPATED LOOSE

EXACERBATING CONDITIONS

CURENT WEATHER

SUNNY OVERCAST

FOGGY

RAINY SNOWY

CURRENT WEATHER AFFECTING ME

1 2 3 4 5 6 7 8 9 10

NONE GREATLY

JOB STRESS LEVEL

1 2 3 4 5 6 7 8 9 10

LOW HIGH

TEMPERATURE

LOW HIGH

FAMILY HOME LIFE STRESS LEVEL

1 2 3 4 5 6 7 8 9 10

LOW HIGH

TOP 3 THINGS I WILL DO TO MY CARE-SELF TODAY

TOP 3 THINGS TO ACCOMPLISH TODAY

TOP 3 HIGHLIGHTS OF MY DAY

NOTES /COMMENTS

DATE: .... DAY: ....

DAILY QUOTE

"..
...."

	AM	PM
WEIGHT		
TEMPERATURE		
BLOOD PRESSURE		

SUGAR LEVEL

BEFORE BREAKFAST :	AFTER BREAKFAST:
BEFORE LUNCH :	AFTER LUNCH :
BEFORE DINNER :	AFTER DINNER :

BEDTIME :

SLEEP LAST NIGHT

/HOURS

NAPS TODAY

/TOTAL HOURS /HOW MANY

DRUGS/VITAMINS /HERBS/MEDICATIONS	REASON	DOSAGE	TIME			REACTION

SYMPTOM NOTES

RECURRING SYMPTOMS	
NEW SYMPTOMS	

PAIN SITE IDENTIFICATION

MARK PAINFUL AREAS OF THE BODY

OVERALL MORNING PAIN LEVEL

1 2 3 4 5 6 7 8 9 10

LOW HIGH

OVERALL AFTERNOON PAIN LEVEL

1 2 3 4 5 6 7 8 9 10

LOW HIGH

OVERALL EVENING PAIN LEVEL

1 2 3 4 5 6 7 8 9 10

LOW HIGH

SUSPECTED TRIGGERS

....
....

MEDICATIONS: ....

DID THE MEDICATION HELP? ....

PHYSICAL ACTIVITY

ACTIVITY/ EXERCISE	DURATION	SETS	REPS	CAL	NOTES

FATIGUE

1 2 3 4 5 6 7 8 9 10

DEPRESSION / ANXIETY

1 2 3 4 5 6 7 8 9 10

MOOD

☆☆☆☆☆

TODAY'S DIET

WATER INTAKE

BREAKFAST TIME :

CAL : CARBS: PROTEIN FAT

LUNCH TIME :

CAL : CARBS: PROTEIN FAT

DINNER TIME :

CAL : CARBS: PROTEIN FAT

SNACKS TIME:

CAL : CARBS: PROTEIN FAT

REACTION TO FOODS

MEAL :

FOOD :

SYMPTOMS

HOW MY APPETITE AFFECTED ?

1 2 3 4 5 6 7 8 9 10

NOT AFFECTED NO APPETITE

HOW IS MY URINATION

1 2 3 4 5 6 7 8 9 10

GOOD WORST

HOW IS MY BOWELS

1 2 3 4 5 6 7 8 9 10

CONSTIPATED LOOSE

EXACERBATING CONDITIONS

CURENT WEATHER

SUNNY OVERCAST

FOGGY

RAINY SNOWY

CURRENT WEATHER AFFECTING ME

1 2 3 4 5 6 7 8 9 10

NONE GREATLY

JOB STRESS LEVEL

1 2 3 4 5 6 7 8 9 10

LOW HIGH

TEMPERATURE

LOW HIGH

FAMILY HOME LIFE STRESS LEVEL

1 2 3 4 5 6 7 8 9 10

LOW HIGH

TOP 3 THINGS I WILL DO TO MY CARE-SELF TODAY

TOP 3 THINGS TO ACCOMPLISH TODAY

TOP 3 HIGHLIGHTS OF MY DAY

NOTES /COMMENTS

DATE: .... DAY: ....

DAILY QUOTE

" ....
.... "

	AM	PM
WEIGHT		
TEMPERATURE		
BLOOD PRESSURE		

SUGAR LEVEL

BEFORE BREAKFAST :	AFTER BREAKFAST:
BEFORE LUNCH :	AFTER LUNCH :
BEFORE DINNER :	AFTER DINNER :

BEDTIME :

SLEEP LAST NIGHT

☐ /HOURS

☐ ☺ ☐ ☹ ☐ 😫

NAPS TODAY

☐ /TOTAL HOURS ☐ /HOW MANY

DRUGS/VITAMINS /HERBS/MEDICATIONS	REASON	DOSAGE	TIME			REACTION

SYMPTOM NOTES

RECURRING SYMPTOMS	
NEW SYMPTOMS	

PAIN SITE IDENTIFICATION

MARK PAINFUL AREAS OF THE BODY

OVERALL MORNING PAIN LEVEL

1 2 3 4 5 6 7 8 9 10

LOW HIGH

OVERALL AFTERNOON PAIN LEVEL

1 2 3 4 5 6 7 8 9 10

LOW HIGH

OVERALL EVENING PAIN LEVEL

1 2 3 4 5 6 7 8 9 10

LOW HIGH

SUSPECTED TRIGGERS

....
....

MEDICATIONS: ....

DID THE MEDICATION HELP? ....

PHYSICAL ACTIVITY

ACTIVITY/ EXERCISE	DURATION	SETS	REPS	CAL	NOTES

FATIGUE

1 2 3 4 5 6 7 8 9 10

DEPRESSION / ANXIETY

1 2 3 4 5 6 7 8 9 10

MOOD

☆ ☆ ☆ ☆ ☆

TODAY'S DIET

WATER INTAKE

BREAKFAST TIME : ....

....

....

....

....

CAL : .... CARBS: .... PROTEIN .... FAT ....

LUNCH TIME : ....

....

....

....

....

CAL : .... CARBS: .... PROTEIN .... FAT ....

DINNER TIME : ....

....

....

....

....

CAL : .... CARBS: .... PROTEIN .... FAT ....

SNACKS TIME: ....

....

....

....

....

CAL : .... CARBS: .... PROTEIN .... FAT ....

REACTION TO FOODS

MEAL : ....

FOOD : ....

SYMPTOMS

....

....

....

....

....

HOW MY APPETITE AFFECTED ?

1 2 3 4 5 6 7 8 9 10

NOT AFFECTED NO APPETITE

HOW IS MY URINATION

1 2 3 4 5 6 7 8 9 10

GOOD WORST

HOW IS MY BOWELS

1 2 3 4 5 6 7 8 9 10

CONSTIPATED LOOSE

EXACERBATING CONDITIONS

CURENT WEATHER

SUNNY OVERCAST

FOGGY

RAINY SNOWY

CURRENT WEATHER AFFECTING ME

1 2 3 4 5 6 7 8 9 10

NONE GREATLY

JOB STRESS LEVEL

1 2 3 4 5 6 7 8 9 10

LOW HIGH

TEMPERATURE

LOW HIGH

FAMILY HOME LIFE STRESS LEVEL

1 2 3 4 5 6 7 8 9 10

LOW HIGH

TOP 3 THINGS I WILL DO TO MY CARE-SELF TODAY

....

....

....

TOP 3 THINGS TO ACCOMPLISH TODAY

....

....

....

TOP 3 HIGHLIGHTS OF MY DAY

....

....

....

NOTES /COMMENTS

....

....

....

....

DATE: .... DAY: ....

DAILY QUOTE

"..
...."

	AM	PM
WEIGHT		
TEMPERATURE		
BLOOD PRESSURE		

SUGAR LEVEL

BEFORE BREAKFAST :	AFTER BREAKFAST:
BEFORE LUNCH :	AFTER LUNCH :
BEFORE DINNER :	AFTER DINNER :

BEDTIME :

SLEEP LAST NIGHT

☐ /HOURS

☐ ☺ ☐ ☹ ☐

NAPS TODAY

☐ /TOTAL HOURS ☐ /HOW MANY

DRUGS/VITAMINS /HERBS/MEDICATIONS	REASON	DOSAGE	TIME			REACTION

SYMPTOM NOTES

RECURRING SYMPTOMS	
NEW SYMPTOMS	

PAIN SITE IDENTIFICATION

MARK PAINFUL AREAS OF THE BODY

OVERALL MORNING PAIN LEVEL

1 2 3 4 5 6 7 8 9 10

LOW HIGH

OVERALL AFTERNOON PAIN LEVEL

1 2 3 4 5 6 7 8 9 10

LOW HIGH

OVERALL EVENING PAIN LEVEL

1 2 3 4 5 6 7 8 9 10

LOW HIGH

SUSPECTED TRIGGERS

....
....

MEDICATIONS: ....

DID THE MEDICATION HELP? ....

PHYSICAL ACTIVITY

ACTIVITY/ EXERCISE	DURATION	SETS	REPS	CAL	NOTES

FATIGUE

1 2 3 4 5 6 7 8 9 10

DEPRESSION / ANXIETY

1 2 3 4 5 6 7 8 9 10

MOOD

☆☆☆☆☆

TODAY'S DIET

WATER INTAKE

BREAKFAST TIME : ....

CAL : .... CARBS: .... PROTEIN .... FAT ....

LUNCH TIME : ....

CAL : .... CARBS: .... PROTEIN .... FAT ....

DINNER TIME : ....

CAL : .... CARBS: .... PROTEIN .... FAT ....

SNACKS TIME: ....

CAL : .... CARBS: .... PROTEIN .... FAT ....

REACTION TO FOODS

MEAL : ....

FOOD : ....

SYMPTOMS

HOW MY APPETITE AFFECTED ?
1 2 3 4 5 6 7 8 9 10
NOT AFFECTED NO APPETITE

HOW IS MY URINATION
1 2 3 4 5 6 7 8 9 10
GOOD WORST

HOW IS MY BOWELS
1 2 3 4 5 6 7 8 9 10
CONSTIPATED LOOSE

EXACERBATING CONDITIONS

CURENT WEATHER
SUNNY OVERCAST
FOGGY
RAINY SNOWY

CURRENT WEATHER AFFECTING ME
1 2 3 4 5 6 7 8 9 10
NONE GREATLY

JOB STRESS LEVEL
1 2 3 4 5 6 7 8 9 10
LOW HIGH

TEMPERATURE
LOW HIGH

FAMILY HOME LIFE STRESS LEVEL
1 2 3 4 5 6 7 8 9 10
LOW HIGH

TOP 3 THINGS I WILL DO TO MY CARE-SELF TODAY

TOP 3 THINGS TO ACCOMPLISH TODAY

TOP 3 HIGHLIGHTS OF MY DAY

NOTES /COMMENTS

DATE: .... DAY: ....

DAILY QUOTE

"..
...."

	AM	PM
WEIGHT		
TEMPERATURE		
BLOOD PRESSURE		

SUGAR LEVEL

BEFORE BREAKFAST :	AFTER BREAKFAST:
BEFORE LUNCH :	AFTER LUNCH :
BEFORE DINNER :	AFTER DINNER :

BEDTIME :

SLEEP LAST NIGHT

☐ /HOURS

☐ ☐ ☐

NAPS TODAY

☐ /TOTAL HOURS ☐ /HOW MANY

DRUGS/VITAMINS /HERBS/MEDICATIONS	REASON	DOSAGE	TIME			REACTION

SYMPTOM NOTES

RECURRING SYMPTOMS	
NEW SYMPTOMS	

PAIN SITE IDENTIFICATION

MARK PAINFUL AREAS OF THE BODY

OVERALL MORNING PAIN LEVEL

1 2 3 4 5 6 7 8 9 10

LOW HIGH

OVERALL AFTERNOON PAIN LEVEL

1 2 3 4 5 6 7 8 9 10

LOW HIGH

OVERALL EVENING PAIN LEVEL

1 2 3 4 5 6 7 8 9 10

LOW HIGH

SUSPECTED TRIGGERS

....
....

MEDICATIONS: ....

DID THE MEDICATION HELP? ....

PHYSICAL ACTIVITY

ACTIVITY/ EXERCISE	DURATION	SETS	REPS	CAL	NOTES

FATIGUE

1 2 3 4 5 6 7 8 9 10

DEPRESSION / ANXIETY

1 2 3 4 5 6 7 8 9 10

MOOD

☆☆☆☆☆

TODAY'S DIET

WATER INTAKE

BREAKFAST TIME : ....

....
....
....
....

CAL : .... CARBS: .... PROTEIN .... FAT ....

LUNCH TIME : ....

....
....
....
....

CAL : .... CARBS: .... PROTEIN .... FAT ....

DINNER TIME : ....

....
....
....
....

CAL : .... CARBS: .... PROTEIN .... FAT ....

SNACKS TIME: ....

....
....
....
....

CAL : .... CARBS: .... PROTEIN .... FAT ....

REACTION TO FOODS

MEAL : ....

FOOD : ....

SYMPTOMS

....
....
....
....
....

HOW MY APPETITE AFFECTED ?

1 2 3 4 5 6 7 8 9 10

NOT AFFECTED NO APPETITE

HOW IS MY URINATION

1 2 3 4 5 6 7 8 9 10

GOOD WORST

HOW IS MY BOWELS

1 2 3 4 5 6 7 8 9 10

CONSTIPATED LOOSE

EXACERBATING CONDITIONS

CURENT WEATHER

SUNNY OVERCAST

FOGGY

RAINY SNOWY

CURRENT WEATHER AFFECTING ME

1 2 3 4 5 6 7 8 9 10

NONE GREATLY

JOB STRESS LEVEL

1 2 3 4 5 6 7 8 9 10

LOW HIGH

TEMPERATURE

LOW HIGH

FAMILY HOME LIFE STRESS LEVEL

1 2 3 4 5 6 7 8 9 10

LOW HIGH

TOP 3 THINGS I WILL DO TO MY CARE-SELF TODAY

....
....
....

TOP 3 THINGS TO ACCOMPLISH TODAY

....
....
....

TOP 3 HIGHLIGHTS OF MY DAY

....
....
....

NOTES /COMMENTS

....
....
....
....

DATE: .... DAY: ....

DAILY QUOTE

" ....
.... "

	AM	PM
WEIGHT		
TEMPERATURE		
BLOOD PRESSURE		

SUGAR LEVEL

BEFORE BREAKFAST :	AFTER BREAKFAST:
BEFORE LUNCH :	AFTER LUNCH :
BEFORE DINNER :	AFTER DINNER :

BEDTIME :

SLEEP LAST NIGHT

/HOURS

NAPS TODAY

/TOTAL HOURS /HOW MANY

DRUGS/VITAMINS /HERBS/MEDICATIONS	REASON	DOSAGE	TIME			REACTION

SYMPTOM NOTES

RECURRING SYMPTOMS	
NEW SYMPTOMS	

PAIN SITE IDENTIFICATION

MARK PAINFUL AREAS OF THE BODY

OVERALL MORNING PAIN LEVEL

1 2 3 4 5 6 7 8 9 10

LOW HIGH

OVERALL AFTERNOON PAIN LEVEL

1 2 3 4 5 6 7 8 9 10

LOW HIGH

OVERALL EVENING PAIN LEVEL

1 2 3 4 5 6 7 8 9 10

LOW HIGH

SUSPECTED TRIGGERS

....
....

MEDICATIONS: ....

DID THE MEDICATION HELP? ....

PHYSICAL ACTIVITY

ACTIVITY/ EXERCISE	DURATION	SETS	REPS	CAL	NOTES

FATIGUE

1 2 3 4 5 6 7 8 9 10

DEPRESSION / ANXIETY

1 2 3 4 5 6 7 8 9 10

MOOD

☆☆☆☆☆

TODAY'S DIET

WATER INTAKE

BREAKFAST TIME : ....

CAL : .... CARBS: .... PROTEIN .... FAT ....

LUNCH TIME : ....

CAL : .... CARBS: .... PROTEIN .... FAT ....

DINNER TIME : ....

CAL : .... CARBS: .... PROTEIN .... FAT ....

SNACKS TIME: ....

CAL : .... CARBS: .... PROTEIN .... FAT ....

REACTION TO FOODS

MEAL : ....

FOOD : ....

SYMPTOMS

HOW MY APPETITE AFFECTED ?

1 2 3 4 5 6 7 8 9 10

NOT AFFECTED NO APPETITE

HOW IS MY URINATION

1 2 3 4 5 6 7 8 9 10

GOOD WORST

HOW IS MY BOWELS

1 2 3 4 5 6 7 8 9 10

CONSTIPATED LOOSE

EXACERBATING CONDITIONS

CURENT WEATHER

SUNNY OVERCAST

FOGGY

RAINY SNOWY

CURRENT WEATHER AFFECTING ME

1 2 3 4 5 6 7 8 9 10

NONE GREATLY

JOB STRESS LEVEL

1 2 3 4 5 6 7 8 9 10

LOW HIGH

TEMPERATURE

LOW HIGH

FAMILY HOME LIFE STRESS LEVEL

1 2 3 4 5 6 7 8 9 10

LOW HIGH

TOP 3 THINGS I WILL DO TO MY CARE-SELF TODAY

TOP 3 THINGS TO ACCOMPLISH TODAY

TOP 3 HIGHLIGHTS OF MY DAY

NOTES /COMMENTS

DATE: .... DAY: ....

DAILY QUOTE

"..
...."

	AM	PM
WEIGHT		
TEMPERATURE		
BLOOD PRESSURE		

SUGAR LEVEL

BEFORE BREAKFAST :	AFTER BREAKFAST:
BEFORE LUNCH :	AFTER LUNCH :
BEFORE DINNER :	AFTER DINNER :

BEDTIME :

SLEEP LAST NIGHT

☐ /HOURS

☐ ☺ ☐ ☹ ☐

NAPS TODAY

☐ /TOTAL HOURS ☐ /HOW MANY

DRUGS/VITAMINS /HERBS/MEDICATIONS	REASON	DOSAGE	TIME			REACTION

SYMPTOM NOTES

RECURRING SYMPTOMS	
NEW SYMPTOMS	

PAIN SITE IDENTIFICATION

MARK PAINFUL AREAS OF THE BODY

OVERALL MORNING PAIN LEVEL

1 2 3 4 5 6 7 8 9 10

LOW HIGH

OVERALL AFTERNOON PAIN LEVEL

1 2 3 4 5 6 7 8 9 10

LOW HIGH

OVERALL EVENING PAIN LEVEL

1 2 3 4 5 6 7 8 9 10

LOW HIGH

SUSPECTED TRIGGERS

....
....

MEDICATIONS: ....

DID THE MEDICATION HELP? ....

PHYSICAL ACTIVITY

ACTIVITY/ EXERCISE	DURATION	SETS	REPS	CAL	NOTES

FATIGUE

1 2 3 4 5 6 7 8 9 10

DEPRESSION / ANXIETY

1 2 3 4 5 6 7 8 9 10

MOOD

☆☆☆☆☆

TODAY'S DIET

WATER INTAKE

BREAKFAST TIME : ....

....
....
....
....

CAL : .... CARBS: .... PROTEIN .... FAT ....

LUNCH TIME : ....

....
....
....
....

CAL : .... CARBS: .... PROTEIN .... FAT ....

DINNER TIME : ....

....
....
....
....

CAL : .... CARBS: .... PROTEIN .... FAT ....

SNACKS TIME: ....

....
....
....
....

CAL : .... CARBS: .... PROTEIN .... FAT ....

REACTION TO FOODS

MEAL : ....

FOOD : ....

SYMPTOMS

....
....
....
....
....

HOW MY APPETITE AFFECTED ?

1 2 3 4 5 6 7 8 9 10

NOT AFFECTED NO APPETITE

HOW IS MY URINATION

1 2 3 4 5 6 7 8 9 10

GOOD WORST

HOW IS MY BOWELS

1 2 3 4 5 6 7 8 9 10

CONSTIPATED LOOSE

EXACERBATING CONDITIONS

CURENT WEATHER

SUNNY OVERCAST

FOGGY

RAINY SNOWY

CURRENT WEATHER AFFECTING ME

1 2 3 4 5 6 7 8 9 10

NONE GREATLY

JOB STRESS LEVEL

1 2 3 4 5 6 7 8 9 10

LOW HIGH

TEMPERATURE

LOW HIGH

FAMILY HOME LIFE STRESS LEVEL

1 2 3 4 5 6 7 8 9 10

LOW HIGH

TOP 3 THINGS I WILL DO TO MY CARE-SELF TODAY

....
....
....

TOP 3 THINGS TO ACCOMPLISH TODAY

....
....
....

TOP 3 HIGHLIGHTS OF MY DAY

....
....
....

NOTES /COMMENTS

....
....
....
....

DATE: .... DAY: ....

DAILY QUOTE

" ....
.... "

	AM	PM
WEIGHT		
TEMPERATURE		
BLOOD PRESSURE		

SUGAR LEVEL

BEFORE BREAKFAST :	AFTER BREAKFAST:
BEFORE LUNCH :	AFTER LUNCH :
BEFORE DINNER :	AFTER DINNER :
BEDTIME :	

SLEEP LAST NIGHT

☐ /HOURS

☐ ☺ ☐ ☹ ☐

NAPS TODAY

☐ /TOTAL HOURS ☐ /HOW MANY

DRUGS/VITAMINS /HERBS/MEDICATIONS	REASON	DOSAGE	TIME			REACTION

SYMPTOM NOTES

RECURRING SYMPTOMS	
NEW SYMPTOMS	

PAIN SITE IDENTIFICATION

MARK PAINFUL AREAS OF THE BODY

OVERALL MORNING PAIN LEVEL

1 2 3 4 5 6 7 8 9 10

LOW HIGH

OVERALL EVENING PAIN LEVEL

1 2 3 4 5 6 7 8 9 10

LOW HIGH

OVERALL AFTERNOON PAIN LEVEL

1 2 3 4 5 6 7 8 9 10

LOW HIGH

SUSPECTED TRIGGERS

....
....

MEDICATIONS: ....

DID THE MEDICATION HELP? ....

PHYSICAL ACTIVITY

ACTIVITY/ EXERCISE	DURATION	SETS	REPS	CAL	NOTES

FATIGUE

1 2 3 4 5 6 7 8 9 10

DEPRESSION / ANXIETY

1 2 3 4 5 6 7 8 9 10

MOOD

☆☆☆☆☆

TODAY'S DIET

WATER INTAKE

BREAKFAST TIME : ....

CAL : .... CARBS: .... PROTEIN .... FAT ....

LUNCH TIME : ....

CAL : .... CARBS: .... PROTEIN .... FAT ....

DINNER TIME : ....

CAL : .... CARBS: .... PROTEIN .... FAT ....

SNACKS TIME: ....

CAL : .... CARBS: .... PROTEIN .... FAT ....

REACTION TO FOODS

MEAL : ....

FOOD : ....

SYMPTOMS

HOW MY APPETITE AFFECTED ?

1 2 3 4 5 6 7 8 9 10

NOT AFFECTED NO APPETITE

HOW IS MY URINATION

1 2 3 4 5 6 7 8 9 10

GOOD WORST

HOW IS MY BOWELS

1 2 3 4 5 6 7 8 9 10

CONSTIPATED LOOSE

EXACERBATING CONDITIONS

CURENT WEATHER

SUNNY OVERCAST

FOGGY

RAINY SNOWY

CURRENT WEATHER AFFECTING ME

1 2 3 4 5 6 7 8 9 10

NONE GREATLY

JOB STRESS LEVEL

1 2 3 4 5 6 7 8 9 10

LOW HIGH

TEMPERATURE

LOW HIGH

FAMILY HOME LIFE STRESS LEVEL

1 2 3 4 5 6 7 8 9 10

LOW HIGH

TOP 3 THINGS I WILL DO TO MY CARE-SELF TODAY

TOP 3 THINGS TO ACCOMPLISH TODAY

TOP 3 HIGHLIGHTS OF MY DAY

NOTES /COMMENTS

DATE: .... **DAY:** ....

DAILY QUOTE

"
....
....
"

	AM	PM
WEIGHT		
TEMPERATURE		
BLOOD PRESSURE		

SUGAR LEVEL

BEFORE BREAKFAST :	AFTER BREAKFAST:
BEFORE LUNCH :	AFTER LUNCH :
BEFORE DINNER :	AFTER DINNER :

BEDTIME :

SLEEP LAST NIGHT

☐ /HOURS

☐ ☺ ☐ ☹ ☐

NAPS TODAY

☐ /TOTAL HOURS ☐ /HOW MANY

DRUGS/VITAMINS /HERBS/MEDICATIONS	REASON	DOSAGE	TIME			REACTION

SYMPTOM NOTES

RECURRING SYMPTOMS	
NEW SYMPTOMS	

PAIN SITE IDENTIFICATION

MARK PAINFUL AREAS OF THE BODY

OVERALL MORNING PAIN LEVEL

1 2 3 4 5 6 7 8 9 10

LOW HIGH

OVERALL AFTERNOON PAIN LEVEL

1 2 3 4 5 6 7 8 9 10

LOW HIGH

OVERALL EVENING PAIN LEVEL

1 2 3 4 5 6 7 8 9 10

LOW HIGH

SUSPECTED TRIGGERS

....
....

MEDICATIONS: ....

DID THE MEDICATION HELP? ....

PHYSICAL ACTIVITY

ACTIVITY/ EXERCISE	DURATION	SETS	REPS	CAL	NOTES

FATIGUE

1 2 3 4 5 6 7 8 9 10

DEPRESSION / ANXIETY

1 2 3 4 5 6 7 8 9 10

MOOD

☆☆☆☆☆

TODAY'S DIET

WATER INTAKE

BREAKFAST TIME : ....

CAL : .... CARBS: .... PROTEIN .... FAT ....

LUNCH TIME : ....

CAL : .... CARBS: .... PROTEIN .... FAT ....

DINNER TIME : ....

CAL : .... CARBS: .... PROTEIN .... FAT ....

SNACKS TIME: ....

CAL : .... CARBS: .... PROTEIN .... FAT ....

REACTION TO FOODS

MEAL : ....

FOOD : ....

SYMPTOMS

HOW MY APPETITE AFFECTED ?

1 2 3 4 5 6 7 8 9 10

NOT AFFECTED NO APPETITE

HOW IS MY URINATION

1 2 3 4 5 6 7 8 9 10

GOOD WORST

HOW IS MY BOWELS

1 2 3 4 5 6 7 8 9 10

CONSTIPATED LOOSE

EXACERBATING CONDITIONS

CURENT WEATHER

SUNNY OVERCAST

FOGGY

RAINY SNOWY

CURRENT WEATHER AFFECTING ME

1 2 3 4 5 6 7 8 9 10

NONE GREATLY

JOB STRESS LEVEL

1 2 3 4 5 6 7 8 9 10

LOW HIGH

TEMPERATURE

LOW HIGH

FAMILY HOME LIFE STRESS LEVEL

1 2 3 4 5 6 7 8 9 10

LOW HIGH

TOP 3 THINGS I WILL DO TO MY CARE-SELF TODAY

TOP 3 THINGS TO ACCOMPLISH TODAY

TOP 3 HIGHLIGHTS OF MY DAY

NOTES /COMMENTS

DATE: .... DAY: ....

DAILY QUOTE

"..
...."

	AM	PM
WEIGHT		
TEMPERATURE		
BLOOD PRESSURE		

SUGAR LEVEL

BEFORE BREAKFAST :	AFTER BREAKFAST:
BEFORE LUNCH :	AFTER LUNCH :
BEFORE DINNER :	AFTER DINNER :
BEDTIME :	

SLEEP LAST NIGHT

☐ /HOURS

☐ ☺ ☐ ☹ ☐

NAPS TODAY

☐ /TOTAL HOURS ☐ /HOW MANY

DRUGS/VITAMINS /HERBS/MEDICATIONS	REASON	DOSAGE	TIME			REACTION

SYMPTOM NOTES

RECURRING SYMPTOMS	
NEW SYMPTOMS	

PAIN SITE IDENTIFICATION

MARK PAINFUL AREAS OF THE BODY

OVERALL MORNING PAIN LEVEL

1 2 3 4 5 6 7 8 9 10

LOW HIGH

OVERALL AFTERNOON PAIN LEVEL

1 2 3 4 5 6 7 8 9 10

LOW HIGH

OVERALL EVENING PAIN LEVEL

1 2 3 4 5 6 7 8 9 10

LOW HIGH

SUSPECTED TRIGGERS

....
....

MEDICATIONS: ....

DID THE MEDICATION HELP? ....

PHYSICAL ACTIVITY

ACTIVITY/ EXERCISE	DURATION	SETS	REPS	CAL	NOTES

FATIGUE

1 2 3 4 5 6 7 8 9 10

DEPRESSION / ANXIETY

1 2 3 4 5 6 7 8 9 10

MOOD

☆☆☆☆☆

TODAY'S DIET

WATER INTAKE

BREAKFAST TIME : ....

CAL : .... CARBS: .... PROTEIN .... FAT ....

LUNCH TIME : ....

CAL : .... CARBS: .... PROTEIN .... FAT ....

DINNER TIME : ....

CAL : .... CARBS: .... PROTEIN .... FAT ....

SNACKS TIME: ....

CAL : .... CARBS: .... PROTEIN .... FAT ....

REACTION TO FOODS

MEAL : ....

FOOD : ....

SYMPTOMS

HOW MY APPETITE AFFECTED ?

1 2 3 4 5 6 7 8 9 10

NOT AFFECTED NO APPETITE

HOW IS MY URINATION

1 2 3 4 5 6 7 8 9 10

GOOD WORST

HOW IS MY BOWELS

1 2 3 4 5 6 7 8 9 10

CONSTIPATED LOOSE

EXACERBATING CONDITIONS

CURENT WEATHER

SUNNY OVERCAST FOGGY RAINY SNOWY

CURRENT WEATHER AFFECTING ME

1 2 3 4 5 6 7 8 9 10

NONE GREATLY

JOB STRESS LEVEL

1 2 3 4 5 6 7 8 9 10

LOW HIGH

TEMPERATURE

LOW HIGH

FAMILY HOME LIFE STRESS LEVEL

1 2 3 4 5 6 7 8 9 10

LOW HIGH

TOP 3 THINGS I WILL DO TO MY CARE-SELF TODAY

TOP 3 THINGS TO ACCOMPLISH TODAY

TOP 3 HIGHLIGHTS OF MY DAY

NOTES /COMMENTS

DATE: .... DAY: ....

DAILY QUOTE

....

....

	AM	PM
WEIGHT		
TEMPERATURE		
BLOOD PRESSURE		

SUGAR LEVEL

BEFORE BREAKFAST :	AFTER BREAKFAST:
BEFORE LUNCH :	AFTER LUNCH :
BEFORE DINNER :	AFTER DINNER :

BEDTIME :

SLEEP LAST NIGHT

☐ /HOURS

☐ ☺ ☐ ☹ ☐ 😫

NAPS TODAY

☐ /TOTAL HOURS ☐ /HOW MANY

DRUGS/VITAMINS /HERBS/MEDICATIONS	REASON	DOSAGE	TIME			REACTION

SYMPTOM NOTES

RECURRING SYMPTOMS	
NEW SYMPTOMS	

PAIN SITE IDENTIFICATION

MARK PAINFUL AREAS OF THE BODY

OVERALL MORNING PAIN LEVEL

1 2 3 4 5 6 7 8 9 10

LOW HIGH

OVERALL AFTERNOON PAIN LEVEL

1 2 3 4 5 6 7 8 9 10

LOW HIGH

OVERALL EVENING PAIN LEVEL

1 2 3 4 5 6 7 8 9 10

LOW HIGH

SUSPECTED TRIGGERS

....

....

MEDICATIONS: ....

DID THE MEDICATION HELP? ....

PHYSICAL ACTIVITY

ACTIVITY/ EXERCISE	DURATION	SETS	REPS	CAL	NOTES

FATIGUE

1 2 3 4 5 6 7 8 9 10

DEPRESSION / ANXIETY

1 2 3 4 5 6 7 8 9 10

MOOD

☆☆☆☆☆

TODAY'S DIET

WATER INTAKE

BREAKFAST TIME : ....

CAL : .... CARBS: .... PROTEIN .... FAT ....

LUNCH TIME : ....

CAL : .... CARBS: .... PROTEIN .... FAT ....

DINNER TIME : ....

CAL : .... CARBS: .... PROTEIN .... FAT ....

SNACKS TIME: ....

CAL : .... CARBS: .... PROTEIN .... FAT ....

REACTION TO FOODS

MEAL : ....

FOOD : ....

SYMPTOMS

HOW MY APPETITE AFFECTED ?

1 2 3 4 5 6 7 8 9 10

NOT AFFECTED NO APPETITE

HOW IS MY URINATION

1 2 3 4 5 6 7 8 9 10

GOOD WORST

HOW IS MY BOWELS

1 2 3 4 5 6 7 8 9 10

CONSTIPATED LOOSE

EXACERBATING CONDITIONS

CURENT WEATHER

SUNNY OVERCAST FOGGY RAINY SNOWY

CURRENT WEATHER AFFECTING ME

1 2 3 4 5 6 7 8 9 10

NONE GREATLY

JOB STRESS LEVEL

1 2 3 4 5 6 7 8 9 10

LOW HIGH

TEMPERATURE

LOW HIGH

FAMILY HOME LIFE STRESS LEVEL

1 2 3 4 5 6 7 8 9 10

LOW HIGH

TOP 3 THINGS I WILL DO TO MY CARE-SELF TODAY

TOP 3 THINGS TO ACCOMPLISH TODAY

TOP 3 HIGHLIGHTS OF MY DAY

NOTES /COMMENTS

DATE: .... **DAY:** ....

DAILY QUOTE

"..

...."

	AM	PM
WEIGHT		
TEMPERATURE		
BLOOD PRESSURE		

SUGAR LEVEL

BEFORE BREAKFAST :	AFTER BREAKFAST:
BEFORE LUNCH :	AFTER LUNCH :
BEFORE DINNER :	AFTER DINNER :

BEDTIME :

SLEEP LAST NIGHT

☐ /HOURS

☐ ☺ ☐ ☹ ☐

NAPS TODAY

☐ /TOTAL HOURS ☐ /HOW MANY

DRUGS/VITAMINS /HERBS/MEDICATIONS	REASON	DOSAGE	TIME			REACTION

SYMPTOM NOTES

RECURRING SYMPTOMS	
NEW SYMPTOMS	

PAIN SITE IDENTIFICATION

MARK PAINFUL AREAS OF THE BODY

OVERALL MORNING PAIN LEVEL

1 2 3 4 5 6 7 8 9 10

LOW HIGH

OVERALL AFTERNOON PAIN LEVEL

1 2 3 4 5 6 7 8 9 10

LOW HIGH

OVERALL EVENING PAIN LEVEL

1 2 3 4 5 6 7 8 9 10

LOW HIGH

SUSPECTED TRIGGERS

....

....

MEDICATIONS: ....

DID THE MEDICATION HELP? ....

PHYSICAL ACTIVITY

ACTIVITY/ EXERCISE	DURATION	SETS	REPS	CAL	NOTES

FATIGUE

1 2 3 4 5 6 7 8 9 10

DEPRESSION / ANXIETY

1 2 3 4 5 6 7 8 9 10

MOOD

☆☆☆☆☆

TODAY'S DIET

WATER INTAKE

BREAKFAST TIME : ....

CAL : .... CARBS: .... PROTEIN .... FAT ....

LUNCH TIME : ....

CAL : .... CARBS: .... PROTEIN .... FAT ....

DINNER TIME : ....

CAL : .... CARBS: .... PROTEIN .... FAT ....

SNACKS TIME: ....

CAL : .... CARBS: .... PROTEIN .... FAT ....

REACTION TO FOODS

MEAL : ....

FOOD : ....

SYMPTOMS

HOW MY APPETITE AFFECTED ?

1 2 3 4 5 6 7 8 9 10

NOT AFFECTED NO APPETITE

HOW IS MY URINATION

1 2 3 4 5 6 7 8 9 10

GOOD WORST

HOW IS MY BOWELS

1 2 3 4 5 6 7 8 9 10

CONSTIPATED LOOSE

EXACERBATING CONDITIONS

CURENT WEATHER

SUNNY OVERCAST

FOGGY

RAINY SNOWY

CURRENT WEATHER AFFECTING ME

1 2 3 4 5 6 7 8 9 10

NONE GREATLY

JOB STRESS LEVEL

1 2 3 4 5 6 7 8 9 10

LOW HIGH

TEMPERATURE

LOW HIGH

FAMILY HOME LIFE STRESS LEVEL

1 2 3 4 5 6 7 8 9 10

LOW HIGH

TOP 3 THINGS I WILL DO TO MY CARE-SELF TODAY

TOP 3 THINGS TO ACCOMPLISH TODAY

TOP 3 HIGHLIGHTS OF MY DAY

NOTES /COMMENTS

DATE: .... DAY: ....

DAILY QUOTE

"..
...."

	AM	PM
WEIGHT		
TEMPERATURE		
BLOOD PRESSURE		

SUGAR LEVEL

BEFORE BREAKFAST :	AFTER BREAKFAST:
BEFORE LUNCH :	AFTER LUNCH :
BEFORE DINNER :	AFTER DINNER :

BEDTIME :

SLEEP LAST NIGHT

☐ /HOURS

☐ ☺ ☐ ☹ ☐

NAPS TODAY

☐ /TOTAL HOURS ☐ /HOW MANY

DRUGS/VITAMINS /HERBS/MEDICATIONS	REASON	DOSAGE	TIME			REACTION

SYMPTOM NOTES

RECURRING SYMPTOMS	
NEW SYMPTOMS	

PAIN SITE IDENTIFICATION

MARK PAINFUL AREAS OF THE BODY

OVERALL MORNING PAIN LEVEL

1 2 3 4 5 6 7 8 9 10

LOW HIGH

OVERALL AFTERNOON PAIN LEVEL

1 2 3 4 5 6 7 8 9 10

LOW HIGH

OVERALL EVENING PAIN LEVEL

1 2 3 4 5 6 7 8 9 10

LOW HIGH

SUSPECTED TRIGGERS

....
....

MEDICATIONS: ....

DID THE MEDICATION HELP? ....

PHYSICAL ACTIVITY

ACTIVITY/ EXERCISE	DURATION	SETS	REPS	CAL	NOTES

FATIGUE

1 2 3 4 5 6 7 8 9 10

DEPRESSION / ANXIETY

1 2 3 4 5 6 7 8 9 10

MOOD

☆☆☆☆☆

TODAY'S DIET

WATER INTAKE

BREAKFAST TIME : ....

CAL : .... CARBS: .... PROTEIN .... FAT ....

LUNCH TIME : ....

CAL : .... CARBS: .... PROTEIN .... FAT ....

DINNER TIME : ....

CAL : .... CARBS: .... PROTEIN .... FAT ....

SNACKS TIME: ....

CAL : .... CARBS: .... PROTEIN .... FAT ....

REACTION TO FOODS

MEAL : ....

FOOD : ....

SYMPTOMS

....

HOW MY APPETITE AFFECTED ?

1 2 3 4 5 6 7 8 9 10

NOT AFFECTED NO APPETITE

HOW IS MY URINATION

1 2 3 4 5 6 7 8 9 10

GOOD WORST

HOW IS MY BOWELS

1 2 3 4 5 6 7 8 9 10

CONSTIPATED LOOSE

EXACERBATING CONDITIONS

CURENT WEATHER

SUNNY OVERCAST

FOGGY

RAINY SNOWY

CURRENT WEATHER AFFECTING ME

1 2 3 4 5 6 7 8 9 10

NONE GREATLY

JOB STRESS LEVEL

1 2 3 4 5 6 7 8 9 10

LOW HIGH

TEMPERATURE

LOW HIGH

FAMILY HOME LIFE STRESS LEVEL

1 2 3 4 5 6 7 8 9 10

LOW HIGH

TOP 3 THINGS I WILL DO TO MY CARE-SELF TODAY

....

TOP 3 THINGS TO ACCOMPLISH TODAY

....

TOP 3 HIGHLIGHTS OF MY DAY

....

NOTES /COMMENTS

....

DATE: .... DAY: ....

DAILY QUOTE

"..
...."

	AM	PM
WEIGHT		
TEMPERATURE		
BLOOD PRESSURE		

SUGAR LEVEL

BEFORE BREAKFAST :	AFTER BREAKFAST:
BEFORE LUNCH :	AFTER LUNCH :
BEFORE DINNER :	AFTER DINNER :

BEDTIME :

SLEEP LAST NIGHT

☐ /HOURS

☐ ☺ ☐ ☹ ☐

NAPS TODAY

☐ /TOTAL HOURS ☐ /HOW MANY

DRUGS/VITAMINS /HERBS/MEDICATIONS	REASON	DOSAGE	TIME			REACTION

SYMPTOM NOTES

RECURRING SYMPTOMS	
NEW SYMPTOMS	

PAIN SITE IDENTIFICATION

MARK PAINFUL AREAS OF THE BODY

OVERALL MORNING PAIN LEVEL

1 2 3 4 5 6 7 8 9 10

LOW HIGH

OVERALL AFTERNOON PAIN LEVEL

1 2 3 4 5 6 7 8 9 10

LOW HIGH

OVERALL EVENING PAIN LEVEL

1 2 3 4 5 6 7 8 9 10

LOW HIGH

SUSPECTED TRIGGERS

....
....

MEDICATIONS: ....

DID THE MEDICATION HELP? ....

PHYSICAL ACTIVITY

ACTIVITY/ EXERCISE	DURATION	SETS	REPS	CAL	NOTES

FATIGUE

1 2 3 4 5 6 7 8 9 10

DEPRESSION / ANXIETY

1 2 3 4 5 6 7 8 9 10

MOOD

☆☆☆☆☆

TODAY'S DIET

WATER INTAKE

BREAKFAST TIME : ....

....

....

....

CAL : .... CARBS: .... PROTEIN .... FAT ....

LUNCH TIME : ....

....

....

....

....

CAL : .... CARBS: .... PROTEIN .... FAT ....

DINNER TIME : ....

....

....

....

....

CAL : .... CARBS: .... PROTEIN .... FAT ....

SNACKS TIME: ....

....

....

....

....

CAL : .... CARBS: .... PROTEIN .... FAT ....

REACTION TO FOODS

MEAL : ....

FOOD : ....

SYMPTOMS

....

....

....

....

....

HOW MY APPETITE AFFECTED ?

1 2 3 4 5 6 7 8 9 10

NOT AFFECTED — NO APPETITE

HOW IS MY URINATION

1 2 3 4 5 6 7 8 9 10

GOOD — WORST

HOW IS MY BOWELS

1 2 3 4 5 6 7 8 9 10

CONSTIPATED — LOOSE

EXACERBATING CONDITIONS

CURENT WEATHER

SUNNY OVERCAST

FOGGY

RAINY SNOWY

CURRENT WEATHER AFFECTING ME

1 2 3 4 5 6 7 8 9 10

NONE — GREATLY

JOB STRESS LEVEL

1 2 3 4 5 6 7 8 9 10

LOW — HIGH

TEMPERATURE

LOW — HIGH

FAMILY HOME LIFE STRESS LEVEL

1 2 3 4 5 6 7 8 9 10

LOW — HIGH

TOP 3 THINGS I WILL DO TO MY CARE-SELF TODAY

....

....

....

TOP 3 THINGS TO ACCOMPLISH TODAY

....

....

....

TOP 3 HIGHLIGHTS OF MY DAY

....

....

....

NOTES /COMMENTS

....

....

....

....

DATE: .... DAY: ....

DAILY QUOTE

" ....
.... "

	AM	PM
WEIGHT		
TEMPERATURE		
BLOOD PRESSURE		

SUGAR LEVEL

BEFORE BREAKFAST :	AFTER BREAKFAST:
BEFORE LUNCH :	AFTER LUNCH :
BEFORE DINNER :	AFTER DINNER :

BEDTIME :

SLEEP LAST NIGHT

☐ /HOURS

☐ ☺ ☐ ☹ ☐

NAPS TODAY

☐ /TOTAL HOURS ☐ /HOW MANY

DRUGS/VITAMINS /HERBS/MEDICATIONS	REASON	DOSAGE	TIME			REACTION

SYMPTOM NOTES

RECURRING SYMPTOMS	
NEW SYMPTOMS	

PAIN SITE IDENTIFICATION

MARK PAINFUL AREAS OF THE BODY

OVERALL MORNING PAIN LEVEL

1 2 3 4 5 6 7 8 9 10

LOW HIGH

OVERALL AFTERNOON PAIN LEVEL

1 2 3 4 5 6 7 8 9 10

LOW HIGH

OVERALL EVENING PAIN LEVEL

1 2 3 4 5 6 7 8 9 10

LOW HIGH

SUSPECTED TRIGGERS

....
....

MEDICATIONS: ....

DID THE MEDICATION HELP? ....

PHYSICAL ACTIVITY

ACTIVITY/ EXERCISE	DURATION	SETS	REPS	CAL	NOTES

FATIGUE

1 2 3 4 5 6 7 8 9 10

DEPRESSION / ANXIETY

1 2 3 4 5 6 7 8 9 10

MOOD

☆☆☆☆☆

TODAY'S DIET

WATER INTAKE

BREAKFAST TIME :

CAL : CARBS: PROTEIN FAT

LUNCH TIME :

CAL : CARBS: PROTEIN FAT

DINNER TIME :

CAL : CARBS: PROTEIN FAT

SNACKS TIME:

CAL : CARBS: PROTEIN FAT

REACTION TO FOODS

MEAL :

FOOD :

SYMPTOMS

HOW MY APPETITE AFFECTED ?

1 2 3 4 5 6 7 8 9 10

NOT AFFECTED NO APPETITE

HOW IS MY URINATION

1 2 3 4 5 6 7 8 9 10

GOOD WORST

HOW IS MY BOWELS

1 2 3 4 5 6 7 8 9 10

CONSTIPATED LOOSE

EXACERBATING CONDITIONS

CURENT WEATHER

SUNNY OVERCAST

FOGGY

RAINY SNOWY

CURRENT WEATHER AFFECTING ME

1 2 3 4 5 6 7 8 9 10

NONE GREATLY

JOB STRESS LEVEL

1 2 3 4 5 6 7 8 9 10

LOW HIGH

TEMPERATURE

LOW HIGH

FAMILY HOME LIFE STRESS LEVEL

1 2 3 4 5 6 7 8 9 10

LOW HIGH

TOP 3 THINGS I WILL DO TO MY CARE-SELF TODAY

TOP 3 THINGS TO ACCOMPLISH TODAY

TOP 3 HIGHLIGHTS OF MY DAY

NOTES /COMMENTS

DATE: .... DAY: ....

DAILY QUOTE

....

....

	AM	PM
WEIGHT		
TEMPERATURE		
BLOOD PRESSURE		

SUGAR LEVEL

BEFORE BREAKFAST :	AFTER BREAKFAST:
BEFORE LUNCH :	AFTER LUNCH :
BEFORE DINNER :	AFTER DINNER :

BEDTIME :

SLEEP LAST NIGHT

/HOURS

NAPS TODAY

/TOTAL HOURS /HOW MANY

DRUGS/VITAMINS /HERBS/MEDICATIONS	REASON	DOSAGE	TIME			REACTION

SYMPTOM NOTES

RECURRING SYMPTOMS	
NEW SYMPTOMS	

PAIN SITE IDENTIFICATION

MARK PAINFUL AREAS OF THE BODY

OVERALL MORNING PAIN LEVEL

1 2 3 4 5 6 7 8 9 10

LOW HIGH

OVERALL AFTERNOON PAIN LEVEL

1 2 3 4 5 6 7 8 9 10

LOW HIGH

OVERALL EVENING PAIN LEVEL

1 2 3 4 5 6 7 8 9 10

LOW HIGH

SUSPECTED TRIGGERS

....

....

MEDICATIONS: ....

DID THE MEDICATION HELP? ....

PHYSICAL ACTIVITY

ACTIVITY/ EXERCISE	DURATION	SETS	REPS	CAL	NOTES

FATIGUE

1 2 3 4 5 6 7 8 9 10

DEPRESSION / ANXIETY

1 2 3 4 5 6 7 8 9 10

MOOD

☆☆☆☆☆

TODAY'S DIET

WATER INTAKE

BREAKFAST TIME : ....

CAL : .... CARBS: .... PROTEIN .... FAT ....

LUNCH TIME : ....

CAL : .... CARBS: .... PROTEIN .... FAT ....

DINNER TIME : ....

CAL : .... CARBS: .... PROTEIN .... FAT ....

SNACKS TIME: ....

CAL : .... CARBS: .... PROTEIN .... FAT ....

REACTION TO FOODS

MEAL : ....

FOOD : ....

SYMPTOMS

HOW MY APPETITE AFFECTED ?

1 2 3 4 5 6 7 8 9 10

NOT AFFECTED NO APPETITE

HOW IS MY URINATION

1 2 3 4 5 6 7 8 9 10

GOOD WORST

HOW IS MY BOWELS

1 2 3 4 5 6 7 8 9 10

CONSTIPATED LOOSE

EXACERBATING CONDITIONS

CURENT WEATHER

SUNNY OVERCAST

FOGGY

RAINY SNOWY

CURRENT WEATHER AFFECTING ME

1 2 3 4 5 6 7 8 9 10

NONE GREATLY

JOB STRESS LEVEL

1 2 3 4 5 6 7 8 9 10

LOW HIGH

TEMPERATURE

LOW HIGH

FAMILY HOME LIFE STRESS LEVEL

1 2 3 4 5 6 7 8 9 10

LOW HIGH

TOP 3 THINGS I WILL DO TO MY CARE-SELF TODAY

TOP 3 THINGS TO ACCOMPLISH TODAY

TOP 3 HIGHLIGHTS OF MY DAY

NOTES /COMMENTS

DATE: .... DAY: ....

DAILY QUOTE

"...
...."

	AM	PM
WEIGHT		
TEMPERATURE		
BLOOD PRESSURE		

SUGAR LEVEL

BEFORE BREAKFAST :	AFTER BREAKFAST:
BEFORE LUNCH :	AFTER LUNCH :
BEFORE DINNER :	AFTER DINNER :

BEDTIME :

SLEEP LAST NIGHT

☐ /HOURS

☐ ☺ ☐ ☹ ☐

NAPS TODAY

☐ /TOTAL HOURS ☐ /HOW MANY

DRUGS/VITAMINS /HERBS/MEDICATIONS	REASON	DOSAGE	TIME			REACTION

SYMPTOM NOTES

RECURRING SYMPTOMS	
NEW SYMPTOMS	

PAIN SITE IDENTIFICATION

MARK PAINFUL AREAS OF THE BODY

OVERALL MORNING PAIN LEVEL

1 2 3 4 5 6 7 8 9 10

LOW HIGH

OVERALL AFTERNOON PAIN LEVEL

1 2 3 4 5 6 7 8 9 10

LOW HIGH

OVERALL EVENING PAIN LEVEL

1 2 3 4 5 6 7 8 9 10

LOW HIGH

SUSPECTED TRIGGERS

....
....

MEDICATIONS: ....

DID THE MEDICATION HELP? ....

PHYSICAL ACTIVITY

ACTIVITY/ EXERCISE	DURATION	SETS	REPS	CAL	NOTES

FATIGUE

1 2 3 4 5 6 7 8 9 10

DEPRESSION / ANXIETY

1 2 3 4 5 6 7 8 9 10

MOOD

☆☆☆☆☆

TODAY'S DIET

WATER INTAKE

BREAKFAST TIME : ....

CAL : .... CARBS: .... PROTEIN .... FAT ....

LUNCH TIME : ....

CAL : .... CARBS: .... PROTEIN .... FAT ....

DINNER TIME : ....

CAL : .... CARBS: .... PROTEIN .... FAT ....

SNACKS TIME: ....

CAL : .... CARBS: .... PROTEIN .... FAT ....

REACTION TO FOODS

MEAL : ....

FOOD : ....

SYMPTOMS

HOW MY APPETITE AFFECTED ?
1 2 3 4 5 6 7 8 9 10
NOT AFFECTED NO APPETITE

HOW IS MY URINATION
1 2 3 4 5 6 7 8 9 10
GOOD WORST

HOW IS MY BOWELS
1 2 3 4 5 6 7 8 9 10
CONSTIPATED LOOSE

EXACERBATING CONDITIONS

CURENT WEATHER
SUNNY OVERCAST
FOGGY
RAINY SNOWY

CURRENT WEATHER AFFECTING ME
1 2 3 4 5 6 7 8 9 10
NONE GREATLY

JOB STRESS LEVEL
1 2 3 4 5 6 7 8 9 10
LOW HIGH

TEMPERATURE
LOW HIGH

FAMILY HOME LIFE STRESS LEVEL
1 2 3 4 5 6 7 8 9 10
LOW HIGH

TOP 3 THINGS I WILL DO TO MY CARE-SELF TODAY

TOP 3 THINGS TO ACCOMPLISH TODAY

TOP 3 HIGHLIGHTS OF MY DAY

NOTES /COMMENTS

DATE:.................. DAY: ....

DAILY QUOTE

"..
...."

	AM	PM
WEIGHT		
TEMPERATURE		
BLOOD PRESSURE		

SUGAR LEVEL

BEFORE BREAKFAST :	AFTER BREAKFAST:
BEFORE LUNCH :	AFTER LUNCH :
BEFORE DINNER :	AFTER DINNER :

BEDTIME :

SLEEP LAST NIGHT

/HOURS

NAPS TODAY

/TOTAL HOURS   /HOW MANY

DRUGS/VITAMINS /HERBS/MEDICATIONS	REASON	DOSAGE	TIME			REACTION

SYMPTOM NOTES

RECURRING SYMPTOMS	
NEW SYMPTOMS	

PAIN SITE IDENTIFICATION

MARK PAINFUL AREAS OF THE BODY

OVERALL MORNING PAIN LEVEL

1 2 3 4 5 6 7 8 9 10

LOW HIGH

OVERALL AFTERNOON PAIN LEVEL

1 2 3 4 5 6 7 8 9 10

LOW HIGH

OVERALL EVENING PAIN LEVEL

1 2 3 4 5 6 7 8 9 10

LOW HIGH

SUSPECTED TRIGGERS

....
....

MEDICATIONS: ....

DID THE MEDICATION HELP? ....

PHYSICAL ACTIVITY

ACTIVITY/ EXERCISE	DURATION	SETS	REPS	CAL	NOTES

FATIGUE

1 2 3 4 5 6 7 8 9 10

DEPRESSION / ANXIETY

1 2 3 4 5 6 7 8 9 10

MOOD

☆☆☆☆☆

TODAY'S DIET

WATER INTAKE

BREAKFAST TIME :

CAL : CARBS: PROTEIN FAT

LUNCH TIME :

CAL : CARBS: PROTEIN FAT

DINNER TIME :

CAL : CARBS: PROTEIN FAT

SNACKS TIME:

CAL : CARBS: PROTEIN FAT

REACTION TO FOODS

MEAL :

FOOD :

SYMPTOMS

HOW MY APPETITE AFFECTED ?

1 2 3 4 5 6 7 8 9 10

NOT AFFECTED NO APPETITE

HOW IS MY URINATION

1 2 3 4 5 6 7 8 9 10

GOOD WORST

HOW IS MY BOWELS

1 2 3 4 5 6 7 8 9 10

CONSTIPATED LOOSE

EXACERBATING CONDITIONS

CURENT WEATHER

SUNNY OVERCAST

FOGGY

RAINY SNOWY

CURRENT WEATHER AFFECTING ME

1 2 3 4 5 6 7 8 9 10

NONE GREATLY

JOB STRESS LEVEL

1 2 3 4 5 6 7 8 9 10

LOW HIGH

TEMPERATURE

LOW HIGH

FAMILY HOME LIFE STRESS LEVEL

1 2 3 4 5 6 7 8 9 10

LOW HIGH

TOP 3 THINGS I WILL DO TO MY CARE-SELF TODAY

TOP 3 THINGS TO ACCOMPLISH TODAY

TOP 3 HIGHLIGHTS OF MY DAY

NOTES /COMMENTS

DATE: .... DAY: ....

DAILY QUOTE

" ....
.... "

	AM	PM
WEIGHT		
TEMPERATURE		
BLOOD PRESSURE		

SUGAR LEVEL

BEFORE BREAKFAST :	AFTER BREAKFAST:
BEFORE LUNCH :	AFTER LUNCH :
BEFORE DINNER :	AFTER DINNER :

BEDTIME :

SLEEP LAST NIGHT

☐ /HOURS

☐ ☺ ☐ ☹ ☐ 😫

NAPS TODAY

☐ /TOTAL HOURS ☐ /HOW MANY

DRUGS/VITAMINS /HERBS/MEDICATIONS	REASON	DOSAGE	TIME			REACTION

SYMPTOM NOTES

RECURRING SYMPTOMS	
NEW SYMPTOMS	

PAIN SITE IDENTIFICATION

MARK PAINFUL AREAS OF THE BODY

OVERALL MORNING PAIN LEVEL

1 2 3 4 5 6 7 8 9 10

LOW HIGH

OVERALL AFTERNOON PAIN LEVEL

1 2 3 4 5 6 7 8 9 10

LOW HIGH

OVERALL EVENING PAIN LEVEL

1 2 3 4 5 6 7 8 9 10

LOW HIGH

SUSPECTED TRIGGERS

....
....

MEDICATIONS: ....

DID THE MEDICATION HELP? ....

PHYSICAL ACTIVITY

ACTIVITY/ EXERCISE	DURATION	SETS	REPS	CAL	NOTES

FATIGUE

1 2 3 4 5 6 7 8 9 10

DEPRESSION / ANXIETY

1 2 3 4 5 6 7 8 9 10

MOOD

☆ ☆ ☆ ☆ ☆

TODAY'S DIET

WATER INTAKE

BREAKFAST TIME : ....

CAL : .... CARBS: .... PROTEIN .... FAT ....

LUNCH TIME : ....

CAL : .... CARBS: .... PROTEIN .... FAT ....

DINNER TIME : ....

CAL : .... CARBS: .... PROTEIN .... FAT ....

SNACKS TIME: ....

CAL : .... CARBS: .... PROTEIN .... FAT ....

REACTION TO FOODS

MEAL : ....

FOOD : ....

SYMPTOMS

HOW MY APPETITE AFFECTED ?

1 2 3 4 5 6 7 8 9 10

NOT AFFECTED NO APPETITE

HOW IS MY URINATION

1 2 3 4 5 6 7 8 9 10

GOOD WORST

HOW IS MY BOWELS

1 2 3 4 5 6 7 8 9 10

CONSTIPATED LOOSE

EXACERBATING CONDITIONS

CURENT WEATHER

SUNNY OVERCAST

FOGGY

RAINY SNOWY

CURRENT WEATHER AFFECTING ME

1 2 3 4 5 6 7 8 9 10

NONE GREATLY

JOB STRESS LEVEL

1 2 3 4 5 6 7 8 9 10

LOW HIGH

TEMPERATURE

LOW HIGH

FAMILY HOME LIFE STRESS LEVEL

1 2 3 4 5 6 7 8 9 10

LOW HIGH

TOP 3 THINGS I WILL DO TO MY CARE-SELF TODAY

TOP 3 THINGS TO ACCOMPLISH TODAY

TOP 3 HIGHLIGHTS OF MY DAY

NOTES /COMMENTS

DATE: .... DAY: ....

DAILY QUOTE

"..
...."

	AM	PM
WEIGHT		
TEMPERATURE		
BLOOD PRESSURE		

SUGAR LEVEL

BEFORE BREAKFAST :	AFTER BREAKFAST:
BEFORE LUNCH :	AFTER LUNCH :
BEFORE DINNER :	AFTER DINNER :

BEDTIME :

SLEEP LAST NIGHT

☐ /HOURS

☐ ☺ ☐ ☹ ☐

NAPS TODAY

☐ /TOTAL HOURS ☐ /HOW MANY

DRUGS/VITAMINS /HERBS/MEDICATIONS	REASON	DOSAGE	TIME			REACTION

SYMPTOM NOTES

RECURRING SYMPTOMS	
NEW SYMPTOMS	

PAIN SITE IDENTIFICATION

MARK PAINFUL AREAS OF THE BODY

OVERALL MORNING PAIN LEVEL

1 2 3 4 5 6 7 8 9 10

LOW HIGH

OVERALL AFTERNOON PAIN LEVEL

1 2 3 4 5 6 7 8 9 10

LOW HIGH

OVERALL EVENING PAIN LEVEL

1 2 3 4 5 6 7 8 9 10

LOW HIGH

SUSPECTED TRIGGERS

....
....

MEDICATIONS: ....

DID THE MEDICATION HELP? ....

PHYSICAL ACTIVITY

ACTIVITY/ EXERCISE	DURATION	SETS	REPS	CAL	NOTES

FATIGUE

1 2 3 4 5 6 7 8 9 10

DEPRESSION / ANXIETY

1 2 3 4 5 6 7 8 9 10

MOOD

☆☆☆☆☆

TODAY'S DIET

WATER INTAKE

BREAKFAST TIME : ....

CAL : .... CARBS: .... PROTEIN .... FAT ....

LUNCH TIME : ....

CAL : .... CARBS: .... PROTEIN .... FAT ....

DINNER TIME : ....

CAL : .... CARBS: .... PROTEIN .... FAT ....

SNACKS TIME: ....

CAL : .... CARBS: .... PROTEIN .... FAT ....

REACTION TO FOODS

MEAL : ....

FOOD : ....

SYMPTOMS

HOW MY APPETITE AFFECTED ?
1 2 3 4 5 6 7 8 9 10
NOT AFFECTED NO APPETITE

HOW IS MY URINATION
1 2 3 4 5 6 7 8 9 10
GOOD WORST

HOW IS MY BOWELS
1 2 3 4 5 6 7 8 9 10
CONSTIPATED LOOSE

EXACERBATING CONDITIONS

CURENT WEATHER
SUNNY OVERCAST
FOGGY
RAINY SNOWY

CURRENT WEATHER AFFECTING ME
1 2 3 4 5 6 7 8 9 10
NONE GREATLY

JOB STRESS LEVEL
1 2 3 4 5 6 7 8 9 10
LOW HIGH

TEMPERATURE
LOW HIGH

FAMILY HOME LIFE STRESS LEVEL
1 2 3 4 5 6 7 8 9 10
LOW HIGH

TOP 3 THINGS I WILL DO TO MY CARE-SELF TODAY

TOP 3 THINGS TO ACCOMPLISH TODAY

TOP 3 HIGHLIGHTS OF MY DAY

NOTES /COMMENTS

DATE: .... DAY: ....

DAILY QUOTE

" ....
...."

	AM	PM
WEIGHT		
TEMPERATURE		
BLOOD PRESSURE		

SUGAR LEVEL

BEFORE BREAKFAST :	AFTER BREAKFAST:
BEFORE LUNCH :	AFTER LUNCH :
BEFORE DINNER :	AFTER DINNER :
BEDTIME :	

SLEEP LAST NIGHT

☐ /HOURS

☐ ☺ ☐ ☹ ☐

NAPS TODAY

☐ /TOTAL HOURS ☐ /HOW MANY

DRUGS/VITAMINS /HERBS/MEDICATIONS	REASON	DOSAGE	TIME			REACTION

SYMPTOM NOTES	
RECURRING SYMPTOMS	
NEW SYMPTOMS	

PAIN SITE IDENTIFICATION

MARK PAINFUL AREAS OF THE BODY

OVERALL MORNING PAIN LEVEL

1 2 3 4 5 6 7 8 9 10

LOW HIGH

OVERALL AFTERNOON PAIN LEVEL

1 2 3 4 5 6 7 8 9 10

LOW HIGH

OVERALL EVENING PAIN LEVEL

1 2 3 4 5 6 7 8 9 10

LOW HIGH

SUSPECTED TRIGGERS

....
....

MEDICATIONS: ....

DID THE MEDICATION HELP? ....

PHYSICAL ACTIVITY

ACTIVITY/ EXERCISE	DURATION	SETS	REPS	CAL	NOTES

FATIGUE

1 2 3 4 5 6 7 8 9 10

DEPRESSION / ANXIETY

1 2 3 4 5 6 7 8 9 10

MOOD

☆ ☆ ☆ ☆ ☆

TODAY'S DIET

WATER INTAKE

BREAKFAST TIME : ....

CAL : .... CARBS: .... PROTEIN .... FAT ....

LUNCH TIME : ....

CAL : .... CARBS: .... PROTEIN .... FAT ....

DINNER TIME : ....

CAL : .... CARBS: .... PROTEIN .... FAT ....

SNACKS TIME: ....

CAL : .... CARBS: .... PROTEIN .... FAT ....

REACTION TO FOODS

MEAL : ....

FOOD : ....

SYMPTOMS

HOW MY APPETITE AFFECTED ?

1 2 3 4 5 6 7 8 9 10

NOT AFFECTED NO APPETITE

HOW IS MY URINATION

1 2 3 4 5 6 7 8 9 10

GOOD WORST

HOW IS MY BOWELS

1 2 3 4 5 6 7 8 9 10

CONSTIPATED LOOSE

EXACERBATING CONDITIONS

CURENT WEATHER

SUNNY OVERCAST

FOGGY

RAINY SNOWY

CURRENT WEATHER AFFECTING ME

1 2 3 4 5 6 7 8 9 10

NONE GREATLY

JOB STRESS LEVEL

1 2 3 4 5 6 7 8 9 10

LOW HIGH

TEMPERATURE

LOW HIGH

FAMILY HOME LIFE STRESS LEVEL

1 2 3 4 5 6 7 8 9 10

LOW HIGH

TOP 3 THINGS I WILL DO TO MY CARE-SELF TODAY

TOP 3 THINGS TO ACCOMPLISH TODAY

TOP 3 HIGHLIGHTS OF MY DAY

NOTES /COMMENTS

DATE: .... DAY: ....

DAILY QUOTE

" .... "
....

	AM	PM
WEIGHT		
TEMPERATURE		
BLOOD PRESSURE		

SUGAR LEVEL

BEFORE BREAKFAST :	AFTER BREAKFAST:
BEFORE LUNCH :	AFTER LUNCH :
BEFORE DINNER :	AFTER DINNER :

BEDTIME :

SLEEP LAST NIGHT

☐ /HOURS

☐ ☺ ☐ ☹ ☐

NAPS TODAY

☐ /TOTAL HOURS ☐ /HOW MANY

DRUGS/VITAMINS /HERBS/MEDICATIONS	REASON	DOSAGE	TIME			REACTION

SYMPTOM NOTES

RECURRING SYMPTOMS	
NEW SYMPTOMS	

PAIN SITE IDENTIFICATION

MARK PAINFUL AREAS OF THE BODY

OVERALL MORNING PAIN LEVEL

1 2 3 4 5 6 7 8 9 10

LOW HIGH

OVERALL AFTERNOON PAIN LEVEL

1 2 3 4 5 6 7 8 9 10

LOW HIGH

OVERALL EVENING PAIN LEVEL

1 2 3 4 5 6 7 8 9 10

LOW HIGH

SUSPECTED TRIGGERS

....
....

MEDICATIONS: ....

DID THE MEDICATION HELP? ....

PHYSICAL ACTIVITY

ACTIVITY/ EXERCISE	DURATION	SETS	REPS	CAL	NOTES

FATIGUE

1 2 3 4 5 6 7 8 9 10

DEPRESSION / ANXIETY

1 2 3 4 5 6 7 8 9 10

MOOD

☆☆☆☆☆

TODAY'S DIET

WATER INTAKE

BREAKFAST TIME : ....

CAL : .... CARBS: .... PROTEIN .... FAT ....

LUNCH TIME : ....

CAL : .... CARBS: .... PROTEIN .... FAT ....

DINNER TIME : ....

CAL : .... CARBS: .... PROTEIN .... FAT ....

SNACKS TIME: ....

CAL : .... CARBS: .... PROTEIN .... FAT ....

REACTION TO FOODS

MEAL : ....

FOOD : ....

SYMPTOMS

HOW MY APPETITE AFFECTED ?

1 2 3 4 5 6 7 8 9 10

NOT AFFECTED NO APPETITE

HOW IS MY URINATION

1 2 3 4 5 6 7 8 9 10

GOOD WORST

HOW IS MY BOWELS

1 2 3 4 5 6 7 8 9 10

CONSTIPATED LOOSE

EXACERBATING CONDITIONS

CURENT WEATHER

SUNNY OVERCAST

FOGGY

RAINY SNOWY

CURRENT WEATHER AFFECTING ME

1 2 3 4 5 6 7 8 9 10

NONE GREATLY

JOB STRESS LEVEL

1 2 3 4 5 6 7 8 9 10

LOW HIGH

TEMPERATURE

LOW HIGH

FAMILY HOME LIFE STRESS LEVEL

1 2 3 4 5 6 7 8 9 10

LOW HIGH

TOP 3 THINGS I WILL DO TO MY CARE-SELF TODAY

TOP 3 THINGS TO ACCOMPLISH TODAY

TOP 3 HIGHLIGHTS OF MY DAY

NOTES /COMMENTS

DATE: .... **DAY:** ....

DAILY QUOTE

"..
...."

	AM	PM
WEIGHT		
TEMPERATURE		
BLOOD PRESSURE		

SUGAR LEVEL

BEFORE BREAKFAST :	AFTER BREAKFAST:
BEFORE LUNCH :	AFTER LUNCH :
BEFORE DINNER :	AFTER DINNER :

BEDTIME :

SLEEP LAST NIGHT

☐ /HOURS

☐ ☺ ☐ ☹ ☐

NAPS TODAY

☐ /TOTAL HOURS ☐ /HOW MANY

DRUGS/VITAMINS /HERBS/MEDICATIONS	REASON	DOSAGE	TIME			REACTION

SYMPTOM NOTES

RECURRING SYMPTOMS	
NEW SYMPTOMS	

PAIN SITE IDENTIFICATION

MARK PAINFUL AREAS OF THE BODY

OVERALL MORNING PAIN LEVEL

1 2 3 4 5 6 7 8 9 10

LOW HIGH

OVERALL AFTERNOON PAIN LEVEL

1 2 3 4 5 6 7 8 9 10

LOW HIGH

OVERALL EVENING PAIN LEVEL

1 2 3 4 5 6 7 8 9 10

LOW HIGH

SUSPECTED TRIGGERS

....
....

MEDICATIONS: ....

DID THE MEDICATION HELP? ....

PHYSICAL ACTIVITY

ACTIVITY/ EXERCISE	DURATION	SETS	REPS	CAL	NOTES

FATIGUE

1 2 3 4 5 6 7 8 9 10

DEPRESSION / ANXIETY

1 2 3 4 5 6 7 8 9 10

MOOD

☆ ☆ ☆ ☆ ☆

TODAY'S DIET

WATER INTAKE

BREAKFAST TIME : ....

CAL : .... CARBS: .... PROTEIN .... FAT ....

LUNCH TIME : ....

CAL : .... CARBS: .... PROTEIN .... FAT ....

DINNER TIME : ....

CAL : .... CARBS: .... PROTEIN .... FAT ....

SNACKS TIME: ....

CAL : .... CARBS: .... PROTEIN .... FAT ....

REACTION TO FOODS

MEAL : ....

FOOD : ....

SYMPTOMS

HOW MY APPETITE AFFECTED ?

1 2 3 4 5 6 7 8 9 10

NOT AFFECTED NO APPETITE

HOW IS MY URINATION

1 2 3 4 5 6 7 8 9 10

GOOD WORST

HOW IS MY BOWELS

1 2 3 4 5 6 7 8 9 10

CONSTIPATED LOOSE

EXACERBATING CONDITIONS

CURENT WEATHER

SUNNY OVERCAST

FOGGY

RAINY SNOWY

CURRENT WEATHER AFFECTING ME

1 2 3 4 5 6 7 8 9 10

NONE GREATLY

JOB STRESS LEVEL

1 2 3 4 5 6 7 8 9 10

LOW HIGH

TEMPERATURE

LOW HIGH

FAMILY HOME LIFE STRESS LEVEL

1 2 3 4 5 6 7 8 9 10

LOW HIGH

TOP 3 THINGS I WILL DO TO MY CARE-SELF TODAY

TOP 3 THINGS TO ACCOMPLISH TODAY

TOP 3 HIGHLIGHTS OF MY DAY

NOTES /COMMENTS

DATE: .... DAY: ....

DAILY QUOTE

"..
...."

	AM	PM
WEIGHT		
TEMPERATURE		
BLOOD PRESSURE		

SUGAR LEVEL

BEFORE BREAKFAST :	AFTER BREAKFAST:
BEFORE LUNCH :	AFTER LUNCH :
BEFORE DINNER :	AFTER DINNER :
BEDTIME :	

SLEEP LAST NIGHT

/HOURS

NAPS TODAY

/TOTAL HOURS /HOW MANY

DRUGS/VITAMINS /HERBS/MEDICATIONS	REASON	DOSAGE	TIME			REACTION

SYMPTOM NOTES

RECURRING SYMPTOMS	
NEW SYMPTOMS	

PAIN SITE IDENTIFICATION

MARK PAINFUL AREAS OF THE BODY

OVERALL MORNING PAIN LEVEL

1 2 3 4 5 6 7 8 9 10

LOW HIGH

OVERALL AFTERNOON PAIN LEVEL

1 2 3 4 5 6 7 8 9 10

LOW HIGH

OVERALL EVENING PAIN LEVEL

1 2 3 4 5 6 7 8 9 10

LOW HIGH

SUSPECTED TRIGGERS

....
....

MEDICATIONS: ....

DID THE MEDICATION HELP? ....

PHYSICAL ACTIVITY

ACTIVITY/ EXERCISE	DURATION	SETS	REPS	CAL	NOTES

FATIGUE

1 2 3 4 5 6 7 8 9 10

DEPRESSION / ANXIETY

1 2 3 4 5 6 7 8 9 10

MOOD

☆☆☆☆☆

TODAY'S DIET

WATER INTAKE

BREAKFAST TIME : ....

CAL : .... CARBS: .... PROTEIN .... FAT ....

LUNCH TIME : ....

CAL : .... CARBS: .... PROTEIN .... FAT ....

DINNER TIME : ....

CAL : .... CARBS: .... PROTEIN .... FAT ....

SNACKS TIME: ....

CAL : .... CARBS: .... PROTEIN .... FAT ....

REACTION TO FOODS

MEAL : ....

FOOD : ....

SYMPTOMS

HOW MY APPETITE AFFECTED ?

1 2 3 4 5 6 7 8 9 10

NOT AFFECTED NO APPETITE

HOW IS MY URINATION

1 2 3 4 5 6 7 8 9 10

GOOD WORST

HOW IS MY BOWELS

1 2 3 4 5 6 7 8 9 10

CONSTIPATED LOOSE

EXACERBATING CONDITIONS

CURENT WEATHER

SUNNY OVERCAST

FOGGY

RAINY SNOWY

CURRENT WEATHER AFFECTING ME

1 2 3 4 5 6 7 8 9 10

NONE GREATLY

JOB STRESS LEVEL

1 2 3 4 5 6 7 8 9 10

LOW HIGH

TEMPERATURE

LOW HIGH

FAMILY HOME LIFE STRESS LEVEL

1 2 3 4 5 6 7 8 9 10

LOW HIGH

TOP 3 THINGS I WILL DO TO MY CARE-SELF TODAY

TOP 3 THINGS TO ACCOMPLISH TODAY

TOP 3 HIGHLIGHTS OF MY DAY

NOTES /COMMENTS

DATE: .... DAY: ....

DAILY QUOTE

"..
...."

	AM	PM
WEIGHT		
TEMPERATURE		
BLOOD PRESSURE		

SUGAR LEVEL

BEFORE BREAKFAST :	AFTER BREAKFAST:
BEFORE LUNCH :	AFTER LUNCH :
BEFORE DINNER :	AFTER DINNER :
BEDTIME :	

SLEEP LAST NIGHT

☐ /HOURS

☐ ☺ ☐ ☹ ☐ 😫

NAPS TODAY

☐ /TOTAL HOURS ☐ /HOW MANY

DRUGS/VITAMINS /HERBS/MEDICATIONS	REASON	DOSAGE	TIME			REACTION

SYMPTOM NOTES

RECURRING SYMPTOMS	
NEW SYMPTOMS	

PAIN SITE IDENTIFICATION

MARK PAINFUL AREAS OF THE BODY

OVERALL MORNING PAIN LEVEL

1 2 3 4 5 6 7 8 9 10

LOW HIGH

OVERALL EVENING PAIN LEVEL

1 2 3 4 5 6 7 8 9 10

LOW HIGH

OVERALL AFTERNOON PAIN LEVEL

1 2 3 4 5 6 7 8 9 10

LOW HIGH

SUSPECTED TRIGGERS

....
....

MEDICATIONS: ....

DID THE MEDICATION HELP? ....

PHYSICAL ACTIVITY

ACTIVITY/ EXERCISE	DURATION	SETS	REPS	CAL	NOTES

FATIGUE

1 2 3 4 5 6 7 8 9 10

DEPRESSION / ANXIETY

1 2 3 4 5 6 7 8 9 10

MOOD

☆ ☆ ☆ ☆ ☆

TODAY'S DIET

WATER INTAKE

BREAKFAST TIME : ....

....

CAL : .... CARBS: .... PROTEIN .... FAT ....

LUNCH TIME : ....

....

CAL : .... CARBS: .... PROTEIN .... FAT ....

DINNER TIME : ....

....

CAL : .... CARBS: .... PROTEIN .... FAT ....

SNACKS TIME: ....

....

CAL : .... CARBS: .... PROTEIN .... FAT ....

REACTION TO FOODS

MEAL : ....

FOOD : ....

SYMPTOMS

....

HOW MY APPETITE AFFECTED ?

1 2 3 4 5 6 7 8 9 10

NOT AFFECTED NO APPETITE

HOW IS MY URINATION

1 2 3 4 5 6 7 8 9 10

GOOD WORST

HOW IS MY BOWELS

1 2 3 4 5 6 7 8 9 10

CONSTIPATED LOOSE

EXACERBATING CONDITIONS

CURENT WEATHER

SUNNY OVERCAST FOGGY RAINY SNOWY

CURRENT WEATHER AFFECTING ME

1 2 3 4 5 6 7 8 9 10

NONE GREATLY

JOB STRESS LEVEL

1 2 3 4 5 6 7 8 9 10

LOW HIGH

TEMPERATURE

LOW HIGH

FAMILY HOME LIFE STRESS LEVEL

1 2 3 4 5 6 7 8 9 10

LOW HIGH

TOP 3 THINGS I WILL DO TO MY CARE-SELF TODAY

....

TOP 3 THINGS TO ACCOMPLISH TODAY

....

TOP 3 HIGHLIGHTS OF MY DAY

....

NOTES /COMMENTS

....

DATE: .... DAY: ....

DAILY QUOTE

"..
...."

	AM	PM
WEIGHT		
TEMPERATURE		
BLOOD PRESSURE		

SUGAR LEVEL

BEFORE BREAKFAST :	AFTER BREAKFAST:
BEFORE LUNCH :	AFTER LUNCH :
BEFORE DINNER :	AFTER DINNER :

BEDTIME :

SLEEP LAST NIGHT

☐ /HOURS

☐ ☺ ☐ ☹ ☐ 😫

NAPS TODAY

☐ /TOTAL HOURS ☐ /HOW MANY

DRUGS/VITAMINS /HERBS/MEDICATIONS	REASON	DOSAGE	TIME			REACTION

SYMPTOM NOTES

RECURRING SYMPTOMS	
NEW SYMPTOMS	

PAIN SITE IDENTIFICATION

MARK PAINFUL AREAS OF THE BODY

OVERALL MORNING PAIN LEVEL

1 2 3 4 5 6 7 8 9 10

LOW HIGH

OVERALL AFTERNOON PAIN LEVEL

1 2 3 4 5 6 7 8 9 10

LOW HIGH

OVERALL EVENING PAIN LEVEL

1 2 3 4 5 6 7 8 9 10

LOW HIGH

SUSPECTED TRIGGERS

....
....

MEDICATIONS: ....

DID THE MEDICATION HELP? ....

PHYSICAL ACTIVITY

ACTIVITY/ EXERCISE	DURATION	SETS	REPS	CAL	NOTES

FATIGUE

1 2 3 4 5 6 7 8 9 10

DEPRESSION / ANXIETY

1 2 3 4 5 6 7 8 9 10

MOOD

☆☆☆☆☆

TODAY'S DIET

WATER INTAKE

BREAKFAST TIME :

CAL : CARBS: PROTEIN FAT

LUNCH TIME :

CAL : CARBS: PROTEIN FAT

DINNER TIME :

CAL : CARBS: PROTEIN FAT

SNACKS TIME:

CAL : CARBS: PROTEIN FAT

REACTION TO FOODS

MEAL :

FOOD :

SYMPTOMS

HOW MY APPETITE AFFECTED ?

1 2 3 4 5 6 7 8 9 10

NOT AFFECTED NO APPETITE

HOW IS MY URINATION

1 2 3 4 5 6 7 8 9 10

GOOD WORST

HOW IS MY BOWELS

1 2 3 4 5 6 7 8 9 10

CONSTIPATED LOOSE

EXACERBATING CONDITIONS

CURENT WEATHER

SUNNY OVERCAST FOGGY RAINY SNOWY

CURRENT WEATHER AFFECTING ME

1 2 3 4 5 6 7 8 9 10

NONE GREATLY

JOB STRESS LEVEL

1 2 3 4 5 6 7 8 9 10

LOW HIGH

TEMPERATURE

LOW HIGH

FAMILY HOME LIFE STRESS LEVEL

1 2 3 4 5 6 7 8 9 10

LOW HIGH

TOP 3 THINGS I WILL DO TO MY CARE-SELF TODAY

TOP 3 THINGS TO ACCOMPLISH TODAY

TOP 3 HIGHLIGHTS OF MY DAY

NOTES /COMMENTS

DATE: .... DAY: ....

DAILY QUOTE

"..
...."

	AM	PM
WEIGHT		
TEMPERATURE		
BLOOD PRESSURE		

SUGAR LEVEL

BEFORE BREAKFAST :	AFTER BREAKFAST:
BEFORE LUNCH :	AFTER LUNCH :
BEFORE DINNER :	AFTER DINNER :

BEDTIME :

SLEEP LAST NIGHT

☐ /HOURS

☐ ☺ ☐ ☹ ☐

NAPS TODAY

☐ /TOTAL HOURS ☐ /HOW MANY

DRUGS/VITAMINS /HERBS/MEDICATIONS	REASON	DOSAGE	TIME			REACTION

SYMPTOM NOTES

RECURRING SYMPTOMS	
NEW SYMPTOMS	

PAIN SITE IDENTIFICATION

MARK PAINFUL AREAS OF THE BODY

OVERALL MORNING PAIN LEVEL

1 2 3 4 5 6 7 8 9 10

LOW HIGH

OVERALL AFTERNOON PAIN LEVEL

1 2 3 4 5 6 7 8 9 10

LOW HIGH

OVERALL EVENING PAIN LEVEL

1 2 3 4 5 6 7 8 9 10

LOW HIGH

SUSPECTED TRIGGERS

....
....

MEDICATIONS: ....

DID THE MEDICATION HELP? ....

PHYSICAL ACTIVITY

ACTIVITY/ EXERCISE	DURATION	SETS	REPS	CAL	NOTES

FATIGUE

1 2 3 4 5 6 7 8 9 10

DEPRESSION / ANXIETY

1 2 3 4 5 6 7 8 9 10

MOOD

☆☆☆☆☆

TODAY'S DIET

WATER INTAKE

BREAKFAST TIME : ....

....
....
....
....

CAL : .... CARBS: .... PROTEIN .... FAT ....

LUNCH TIME : ....

....
....
....
....

CAL : .... CARBS: .... PROTEIN .... FAT ....

DINNER TIME : ....

....
....
....
....

CAL : .... CARBS: .... PROTEIN .... FAT ....

SNACKS TIME: ....

....
....
....
....

CAL : .... CARBS: .... PROTEIN .... FAT ....

REACTION TO FOODS

MEAL : ....

FOOD : ....

SYMPTOMS

....
....
....
....
....

HOW MY APPETITE AFFECTED ?

1 2 3 4 5 6 7 8 9 10

NOT AFFECTED NO APPETITE

HOW IS MY URINATION

1 2 3 4 5 6 7 8 9 10

GOOD WORST

HOW IS MY BOWELS

1 2 3 4 5 6 7 8 9 10

CONSTIPATED LOOSE

EXACERBATING CONDITIONS

CURENT WEATHER

SUNNY OVERCAST

FOGGY

RAINY SNOWY

CURRENT WEATHER AFFECTING ME

1 2 3 4 5 6 7 8 9 10

NONE GREATLY

JOB STRESS LEVEL

1 2 3 4 5 6 7 8 9 10

LOW HIGH

TEMPERATURE

LOW HIGH

FAMILY HOME LIFE STRESS LEVEL

1 2 3 4 5 6 7 8 9 10

LOW HIGH

TOP 3 THINGS I WILL DO TO MY CARE-SELF TODAY

....
....
....

TOP 3 THINGS TO ACCOMPLISH TODAY

....
....
....

TOP 3 HIGHLIGHTS OF MY DAY

....
....
....

NOTES /COMMENTS

....
....
....
....

DATE: .... DAY: ....

DAILY QUOTE

....

....

	AM	PM
WEIGHT		
TEMPERATURE		
BLOOD PRESSURE		

SUGAR LEVEL

BEFORE BREAKFAST :	AFTER BREAKFAST:
BEFORE LUNCH :	AFTER LUNCH :
BEFORE DINNER :	AFTER DINNER :

BEDTIME :

SLEEP LAST NIGHT

☐ /HOURS

☐ ☺ ☐ ☹ ☐

NAPS TODAY

☐ /TOTAL HOURS ☐ /HOW MANY

DRUGS/VITAMINS /HERBS/MEDICATIONS	REASON	DOSAGE	TIME			REACTION

SYMPTOM NOTES

RECURRING SYMPTOMS	
NEW SYMPTOMS	

PAIN SITE IDENTIFICATION

MARK PAINFUL AREAS OF THE BODY

OVERALL MORNING PAIN LEVEL

1 2 3 4 5 6 7 8 9 10

LOW HIGH

OVERALL AFTERNOON PAIN LEVEL

1 2 3 4 5 6 7 8 9 10

LOW HIGH

OVERALL EVENING PAIN LEVEL

1 2 3 4 5 6 7 8 9 10

LOW HIGH

SUSPECTED TRIGGERS

....

....

MEDICATIONS: ....

DID THE MEDICATION HELP? ....

PHYSICAL ACTIVITY

ACTIVITY/ EXERCISE	DURATION	SETS	REPS	CAL	NOTES

FATIGUE

1 2 3 4 5 6 7 8 9 10

DEPRESSION / ANXIETY

1 2 3 4 5 6 7 8 9 10

MOOD

☆☆☆☆☆

TODAY'S DIET

WATER INTAKE

BREAKFAST TIME : ....

....
....
....
....

CAL : .... CARBS: .... PROTEIN .... FAT ....

LUNCH TIME : ....

....
....
....
....

CAL : .... CARBS: .... PROTEIN .... FAT ....

DINNER TIME : ....

....
....
....
....

CAL : .... CARBS: .... PROTEIN .... FAT ....

SNACKS TIME: ....

....
....
....
....

CAL : .... CARBS: .... PROTEIN .... FAT ....

REACTION TO FOODS

MEAL : ....

FOOD : ....

SYMPTOMS

....
....
....
....
....

HOW MY APPETITE AFFECTED ?

1 2 3 4 5 6 7 8 9 10

NOT AFFECTED NO APPETITE

HOW IS MY URINATION

1 2 3 4 5 6 7 8 9 10

GOOD WORST

HOW IS MY BOWELS

1 2 3 4 5 6 7 8 9 10

CONSTIPATED LOOSE

EXACERBATING CONDITIONS

CURENT WEATHER

SUNNY OVERCAST

FOGGY

RAINY SNOWY

CURRENT WEATHER AFFECTING ME

1 2 3 4 5 6 7 8 9 10

NONE GREATLY

JOB STRESS LEVEL

1 2 3 4 5 6 7 8 9 10

LOW HIGH

TEMPERATURE

LOW HIGH

FAMILY HOME LIFE STRESS LEVEL

1 2 3 4 5 6 7 8 9 10

LOW HIGH

TOP 3 THINGS I WILL DO TO MY CARE-SELF TODAY

....
....
....

TOP 3 THINGS TO ACCOMPLISH TODAY

....
....
....

TOP 3 HIGHLIGHTS OF MY DAY

....
....
....

NOTES /COMMENTS

....
....
....
....

DATE: .... DAY: ....

DAILY QUOTE

"..
...."

	AM	PM
WEIGHT		
TEMPERATURE		
BLOOD PRESSURE		

SUGAR LEVEL

BEFORE BREAKFAST :	AFTER BREAKFAST:
BEFORE LUNCH :	AFTER LUNCH :
BEFORE DINNER :	AFTER DINNER :
BEDTIME :	

SLEEP LAST NIGHT

☐ /HOURS

☐ ☺ ☐ ☹ ☐ 😫

NAPS TODAY

☐ /TOTAL HOURS ☐ /HOW MANY

DRUGS/VITAMINS /HERBS/MEDICATIONS	REASON	DOSAGE	TIME			REACTION

SYMPTOM NOTES

RECURRING SYMPTOMS	
NEW SYMPTOMS	

PAIN SITE IDENTIFICATION

MARK PAINFUL AREAS OF THE BODY

OVERALL MORNING PAIN LEVEL

1 2 3 4 5 6 7 8 9 10

LOW HIGH

OVERALL EVENING PAIN LEVEL

1 2 3 4 5 6 7 8 9 10

LOW HIGH

OVERALL AFTERNOON PAIN LEVEL

1 2 3 4 5 6 7 8 9 10

LOW HIGH

SUSPECTED TRIGGERS

....
....

MEDICATIONS: ....

DID THE MEDICATION HELP? ....

PHYSICAL ACTIVITY

ACTIVITY/ EXERCISE	DURATION	SETS	REPS	CAL	NOTES

FATIGUE

1 2 3 4 5 6 7 8 9 10

DEPRESSION / ANXIETY

1 2 3 4 5 6 7 8 9 10

MOOD

☆ ☆ ☆ ☆ ☆

TODAY'S DIET

WATER INTAKE

BREAKFAST TIME :

CAL : CARBS: PROTEIN FAT

LUNCH TIME :

CAL : CARBS: PROTEIN FAT

DINNER TIME :

CAL : CARBS: PROTEIN FAT

SNACKS TIME:

CAL : CARBS: PROTEIN FAT

REACTION TO FOODS

MEAL :

FOOD :

SYMPTOMS

HOW MY APPETITE AFFECTED ?

1 2 3 4 5 6 7 8 9 10

NOT AFFECTED NO APPETITE

HOW IS MY URINATION

1 2 3 4 5 6 7 8 9 10

GOOD WORST

HOW IS MY BOWELS

1 2 3 4 5 6 7 8 9 10

CONSTIPATED LOOSE

EXACERBATING CONDITIONS

CURENT WEATHER

SUNNY OVERCAST

FOGGY

RAINY SNOWY

CURRENT WEATHER AFFECTING ME

1 2 3 4 5 6 7 8 9 10

NONE GREATLY

JOB STRESS LEVEL

1 2 3 4 5 6 7 8 9 10

LOW HIGH

TEMPERATURE

LOW HIGH

FAMILY HOME LIFE STRESS LEVEL

1 2 3 4 5 6 7 8 9 10

LOW HIGH

TOP 3 THINGS I WILL DO TO MY CARE-SELF TODAY

TOP 3 THINGS TO ACCOMPLISH TODAY

TOP 3 HIGHLIGHTS OF MY DAY

NOTES /COMMENTS

DATE: .... **DAY:** ....

DAILY QUOTE

"..
...."

	AM	PM
WEIGHT		
TEMPERATURE		
BLOOD PRESSURE		

SUGAR LEVEL

BEFORE BREAKFAST :	AFTER BREAKFAST:
BEFORE LUNCH :	AFTER LUNCH :
BEFORE DINNER :	AFTER DINNER :
BEDTIME :	

SLEEP LAST NIGHT

☐ /HOURS

☐ ☺ ☐ ☹ ☐

NAPS TODAY

☐ /TOTAL HOURS ☐ /HOW MANY

DRUGS/VITAMINS /HERBS/MEDICATIONS	REASON	DOSAGE		TIME		REACTION

SYMPTOM NOTES

RECURRING SYMPTOMS	
NEW SYMPTOMS	

PAIN SITE IDENTIFICATION

MARK PAINFUL AREAS OF THE BODY

OVERALL MORNING PAIN LEVEL

1 2 3 4 5 6 7 8 9 10

LOW HIGH

OVERALL AFTERNOON PAIN LEVEL

1 2 3 4 5 6 7 8 9 10

LOW HIGH

OVERALL EVENING PAIN LEVEL

1 2 3 4 5 6 7 8 9 10

LOW HIGH

SUSPECTED TRIGGERS

....
....

MEDICATIONS: ....

DID THE MEDICATION HELP? ....

PHYSICAL ACTIVITY

ACTIVITY/ EXERCISE	DURATION	SETS	REPS	CAL	NOTES

FATIGUE

1 2 3 4 5 6 7 8 9 10

DEPRESSION / ANXIETY

1 2 3 4 5 6 7 8 9 10

MOOD

☆☆☆☆☆

TODAY'S DIET

WATER INTAKE

BREAKFAST TIME : ....

....
....
....
....

CAL : .... CARBS: .... PROTEIN .... FAT ....

LUNCH TIME : ....

....
....
....
....

CAL : .... CARBS: .... PROTEIN .... FAT ....

DINNER TIME : ....

....
....
....
....

CAL : .... CARBS: .... PROTEIN .... FAT ....

SNACKS TIME: ....

....
....
....
....

CAL : .... CARBS: .... PROTEIN .... FAT ....

REACTION TO FOODS

MEAL : ....

FOOD : ....

SYMPTOMS

....
....
....
....
....

HOW MY APPETITE AFFECTED ?

1 2 3 4 5 6 7 8 9 10

NOT AFFECTED NO APPETITE

HOW IS MY URINATION

1 2 3 4 5 6 7 8 9 10

GOOD WORST

HOW IS MY BOWELS

1 2 3 4 5 6 7 8 9 10

CONSTIPATED LOOSE

EXACERBATING CONDITIONS

CURENT WEATHER

SUNNY OVERCAST

FOGGY

RAINY SNOWY

CURRENT WEATHER AFFECTING ME

1 2 3 4 5 6 7 8 9 10

NONE GREATLY

JOB STRESS LEVEL

1 2 3 4 5 6 7 8 9 10

LOW HIGH

TEMPERATURE

LOW HIGH

FAMILY HOME LIFE STRESS LEVEL

1 2 3 4 5 6 7 8 9 10

LOW HIGH

TOP 3 THINGS I WILL DO TO MY CARE-SELF TODAY

....
....
....

TOP 3 THINGS TO ACCOMPLISH TODAY

....
....
....

TOP 3 HIGHLIGHTS OF MY DAY

....
....
....

NOTES /COMMENTS

....
....
....
....

DATE: .... **DAY:** ....

DAILY QUOTE

"..
...."

	AM	PM
WEIGHT		
TEMPERATURE		
BLOOD PRESSURE		

SUGAR LEVEL

BEFORE BREAKFAST :	AFTER BREAKFAST:
BEFORE LUNCH :	AFTER LUNCH :
BEFORE DINNER :	AFTER DINNER :
BEDTIME :	

SLEEP LAST NIGHT

☐ /HOURS

☐ ☺ ☐ ☹ ☐

NAPS TODAY

☐ /TOTAL HOURS ☐ /HOW MANY

DRUGS/VITAMINS /HERBS/MEDICATIONS	REASON	DOSAGE	TIME			REACTION

SYMPTOM NOTES

RECURRING SYMPTOMS	
NEW SYMPTOMS	

PAIN SITE IDENTIFICATION

MARK PAINFUL AREAS OF THE BODY

OVERALL MORNING PAIN LEVEL

1 2 3 4 5 6 7 8 9 10

LOW HIGH

OVERALL AFTERNOON PAIN LEVEL

1 2 3 4 5 6 7 8 9 10

LOW HIGH

OVERALL EVENING PAIN LEVEL

1 2 3 4 5 6 7 8 9 10

LOW HIGH

SUSPECTED TRIGGERS

....
....

MEDICATIONS: ....

DID THE MEDICATION HELP? ....

PHYSICAL ACTIVITY

ACTIVITY/ EXERCISE	DURATION	SETS	REPS	CAL	NOTES

FATIGUE

1 2 3 4 5 6 7 8 9 10

DEPRESSION / ANXIETY

1 2 3 4 5 6 7 8 9 10

MOOD

☆☆☆☆☆

TODAY'S DIET

WATER INTAKE

BREAKFAST TIME : ....

CAL : .... CARBS: .... PROTEIN .... FAT ....

LUNCH TIME : ....

CAL : .... CARBS: .... PROTEIN .... FAT ....

DINNER TIME : ....

CAL : .... CARBS: .... PROTEIN .... FAT ....

SNACKS TIME: ....

CAL : .... CARBS: .... PROTEIN .... FAT ....

REACTION TO FOODS

MEAL : ....

FOOD : ....

SYMPTOMS

HOW MY APPETITE AFFECTED ?

1 2 3 4 5 6 7 8 9 10

NOT AFFECTED NO APPETITE

HOW IS MY URINATION

1 2 3 4 5 6 7 8 9 10

GOOD WORST

HOW IS MY BOWELS

1 2 3 4 5 6 7 8 9 10

CONSTIPATED LOOSE

EXACERBATING CONDITIONS

CURENT WEATHER

SUNNY OVERCAST

FOGGY

RAINY SNOWY

CURRENT WEATHER AFFECTING ME

1 2 3 4 5 6 7 8 9 10

NONE GREATLY

TEMPERATURE

LOW HIGH

JOB STRESS LEVEL

1 2 3 4 5 6 7 8 9 10

LOW HIGH

FAMILY HOME LIFE STRESS LEVEL

1 2 3 4 5 6 7 8 9 10

LOW HIGH

TOP 3 THINGS I WILL DO TO MY CARE-SELF TODAY

TOP 3 THINGS TO ACCOMPLISH TODAY

TOP 3 HIGHLIGHTS OF MY DAY

NOTES /COMMENTS

DATE: .... DAY: ....

DAILY QUOTE

" ....
.... "

	AM	PM
WEIGHT		
TEMPERATURE		
BLOOD PRESSURE		

SUGAR LEVEL

BEFORE BREAKFAST :	AFTER BREAKFAST:
BEFORE LUNCH :	AFTER LUNCH :
BEFORE DINNER :	AFTER DINNER :

BEDTIME :

SLEEP LAST NIGHT

☐ /HOURS

☐ ☺ ☐ ☹ ☐

NAPS TODAY

☐ /TOTAL HOURS ☐ /HOW MANY

DRUGS/VITAMINS /HERBS/MEDICATIONS	REASON	DOSAGE	TIME			REACTION

SYMPTOM NOTES

RECURRING SYMPTOMS	
NEW SYMPTOMS	

PAIN SITE IDENTIFICATION

MARK PAINFUL AREAS OF THE BODY

OVERALL MORNING PAIN LEVEL

1 2 3 4 5 6 7 8 9 10

LOW HIGH

OVERALL EVENING PAIN LEVEL

1 2 3 4 5 6 7 8 9 10

LOW HIGH

OVERALL AFTERNOON PAIN LEVEL

1 2 3 4 5 6 7 8 9 10

LOW HIGH

SUSPECTED TRIGGERS

....
....

MEDICATIONS: ....

DID THE MEDICATION HELP? ....

PHYSICAL ACTIVITY

ACTIVITY/ EXERCISE	DURATION	SETS	REPS	CAL	NOTES

FATIGUE

1 2 3 4 5 6 7 8 9 10

DEPRESSION / ANXIETY

1 2 3 4 5 6 7 8 9 10

MOOD

☆☆☆☆☆

TODAY'S DIET

WATER INTAKE

BREAKFAST TIME : ....

CAL : .... CARBS: .... PROTEIN .... FAT ....

LUNCH TIME : ....

CAL : .... CARBS: .... PROTEIN .... FAT ....

DINNER TIME : ....

CAL : .... CARBS: .... PROTEIN .... FAT ....

SNACKS TIME: ....

CAL : .... CARBS: .... PROTEIN .... FAT ....

REACTION TO FOODS

MEAL : ....

FOOD : ....

SYMPTOMS

HOW MY APPETITE AFFECTED ?

1 2 3 4 5 6 7 8 9 10

NOT AFFECTED NO APPETITE

HOW IS MY URINATION

1 2 3 4 5 6 7 8 9 10

GOOD WORST

HOW IS MY BOWELS

1 2 3 4 5 6 7 8 9 10

CONSTIPATED LOOSE

EXACERBATING CONDITIONS

CURENT WEATHER

SUNNY OVERCAST

FOGGY

RAINY SNOWY

CURRENT WEATHER AFFECTING ME

1 2 3 4 5 6 7 8 9 10

NONE GREATLY

JOB STRESS LEVEL

1 2 3 4 5 6 7 8 9 10

LOW HIGH

TEMPERATURE

LOW HIGH

FAMILY HOME LIFE STRESS LEVEL

1 2 3 4 5 6 7 8 9 10

LOW HIGH

TOP 3 THINGS I WILL DO TO MY CARE-SELF TODAY

TOP 3 THINGS TO ACCOMPLISH TODAY

TOP 3 HIGHLIGHTS OF MY DAY

NOTES /COMMENTS

DATE: .... DAY: ....

DAILY QUOTE

"..
...."

	AM	PM
WEIGHT		
TEMPERATURE		
BLOOD PRESSURE		

SUGAR LEVEL

BEFORE BREAKFAST :	AFTER BREAKFAST:
BEFORE LUNCH :	AFTER LUNCH :
BEFORE DINNER :	AFTER DINNER :

BEDTIME :

SLEEP LAST NIGHT

☐ /HOURS

☐ ☺ ☐ ☹ ☐

NAPS TODAY

☐ /TOTAL HOURS ☐ /HOW MANY

DRUGS/VITAMINS /HERBS/MEDICATIONS	REASON	DOSAGE	TIME			REACTION

SYMPTOM NOTES

RECURRING SYMPTOMS	
NEW SYMPTOMS	

PAIN SITE IDENTIFICATION

MARK PAINFUL AREAS OF THE BODY

OVERALL MORNING PAIN LEVEL

1 2 3 4 5 6 7 8 9 10

LOW HIGH

OVERALL AFTERNOON PAIN LEVEL

1 2 3 4 5 6 7 8 9 10

LOW HIGH

OVERALL EVENING PAIN LEVEL

1 2 3 4 5 6 7 8 9 10

LOW HIGH

SUSPECTED TRIGGERS

....
....

MEDICATIONS: ....

DID THE MEDICATION HELP? ....

PHYSICAL ACTIVITY

ACTIVITY/ EXERCISE	DURATION	SETS	REPS	CAL	NOTES

FATIGUE

1 2 3 4 5 6 7 8 9 10

DEPRESSION / ANXIETY

1 2 3 4 5 6 7 8 9 10

MOOD

☆☆☆☆☆

TODAY'S DIET

WATER INTAKE

BREAKFAST TIME :

CAL : CARBS: PROTEIN FAT

LUNCH TIME :

CAL : CARBS: PROTEIN FAT

DINNER TIME :

CAL : CARBS: PROTEIN FAT

SNACKS TIME:

CAL : CARBS: PROTEIN FAT

REACTION TO FOODS

MEAL :

FOOD :

SYMPTOMS

HOW MY APPETITE AFFECTED ?

1 2 3 4 5 6 7 8 9 10

NOT AFFECTED NO APPETITE

HOW IS MY URINATION

1 2 3 4 5 6 7 8 9 10

GOOD WORST

HOW IS MY BOWELS

1 2 3 4 5 6 7 8 9 10

CONSTIPATED LOOSE

EXACERBATING CONDITIONS

CURENT WEATHER

SUNNY OVERCAST

FOGGY

RAINY SNOWY

CURRENT WEATHER AFFECTING ME

1 2 3 4 5 6 7 8 9 10

NONE GREATLY

JOB STRESS LEVEL

1 2 3 4 5 6 7 8 9 10

LOW HIGH

TEMPERATURE

LOW HIGH

FAMILY HOME LIFE STRESS LEVEL

1 2 3 4 5 6 7 8 9 10

LOW HIGH

TOP 3 THINGS I WILL DO TO MY CARE-SELF TODAY

TOP 3 THINGS TO ACCOMPLISH TODAY

TOP 3 HIGHLIGHTS OF MY DAY

NOTES /COMMENTS

DATE: .... **DAY:** ....

DAILY QUOTE

"..
...."

	AM	PM
WEIGHT		
TEMPERATURE		
BLOOD PRESSURE		

SUGAR LEVEL

BEFORE BREAKFAST :	AFTER BREAKFAST:
BEFORE LUNCH :	AFTER LUNCH :
BEFORE DINNER :	AFTER DINNER :
BEDTIME :	

SLEEP LAST NIGHT

☐ /HOURS

☐ ☺ ☐ ☹ ☐

NAPS TODAY

☐ /TOTAL HOURS ☐ /HOW MANY

DRUGS/VITAMINS /HERBS/MEDICATIONS	REASON	DOSAGE	TIME			REACTION

SYMPTOM NOTES

RECURRING SYMPTOMS	
NEW SYMPTOMS	

PAIN SITE IDENTIFICATION

MARK PAINFUL AREAS OF THE BODY

OVERALL MORNING PAIN LEVEL

1 2 3 4 5 6 7 8 9 10

LOW HIGH

OVERALL AFTERNOON PAIN LEVEL

1 2 3 4 5 6 7 8 9 10

LOW HIGH

OVERALL EVENING PAIN LEVEL

1 2 3 4 5 6 7 8 9 10

LOW HIGH

SUSPECTED TRIGGERS

....
....

MEDICATIONS: ....

DID THE MEDICATION HELP? ....

PHYSICAL ACTIVITY

ACTIVITY/ EXERCISE	DURATION	SETS	REPS	CAL	NOTES

FATIGUE

1 2 3 4 5 6 7 8 9 10

DEPRESSION / ANXIETY

1 2 3 4 5 6 7 8 9 10

MOOD

☆☆☆☆☆

TODAY'S DIET

WATER INTAKE

BREAKFAST TIME : ....

CAL : .... CARBS: .... PROTEIN .... FAT ....

LUNCH TIME : ....

CAL : .... CARBS: .... PROTEIN .... FAT ....

DINNER TIME : ....

CAL : .... CARBS: .... PROTEIN .... FAT ....

SNACKS TIME: ....

CAL : .... CARBS: .... PROTEIN .... FAT ....

REACTION TO FOODS

MEAL : ....

FOOD : ....

SYMPTOMS

HOW MY APPETITE AFFECTED ?

1 2 3 4 5 6 7 8 9 10

NOT AFFECTED NO APPETITE

HOW IS MY URINATION

1 2 3 4 5 6 7 8 9 10

GOOD WORST

HOW IS MY BOWELS

1 2 3 4 5 6 7 8 9 10

CONSTIPATED LOOSE

EXACERBATING CONDITIONS

CURENT WEATHER

SUNNY OVERCAST

FOGGY

RAINY SNOWY

CURRENT WEATHER AFFECTING ME

1 2 3 4 5 6 7 8 9 10

NONE GREATLY

JOB STRESS LEVEL

1 2 3 4 5 6 7 8 9 10

LOW HIGH

TEMPERATURE

LOW HIGH

FAMILY HOME LIFE STRESS LEVEL

1 2 3 4 5 6 7 8 9 10

LOW HIGH

TOP 3 THINGS I WILL DO TO MY CARE-SELF TODAY

TOP 3 THINGS TO ACCOMPLISH TODAY

TOP 3 HIGHLIGHTS OF MY DAY

NOTES /COMMENTS

DATE: .... DAY: ....

DAILY QUOTE

"..
...."

	AM	PM
WEIGHT		
TEMPERATURE		
BLOOD PRESSURE		

SUGAR LEVEL

BEFORE BREAKFAST :	AFTER BREAKFAST:
BEFORE LUNCH :	AFTER LUNCH :
BEFORE DINNER :	AFTER DINNER :

BEDTIME :

SLEEP LAST NIGHT

☐ /HOURS

☐ ☺ ☐ ☹ ☐

NAPS TODAY

☐ /TOTAL HOURS ☐ /HOW MANY

DRUGS/VITAMINS /HERBS/MEDICATIONS	REASON	DOSAGE	TIME			REACTION

SYMPTOM NOTES

RECURRING SYMPTOMS	
NEW SYMPTOMS	

PAIN SITE IDENTIFICATION

MARK PAINFUL AREAS OF THE BODY

OVERALL MORNING PAIN LEVEL

1 2 3 4 5 6 7 8 9 10

LOW HIGH

OVERALL AFTERNOON PAIN LEVEL

1 2 3 4 5 6 7 8 9 10

LOW HIGH

OVERALL EVENING PAIN LEVEL

1 2 3 4 5 6 7 8 9 10

LOW HIGH

SUSPECTED TRIGGERS

....
....

MEDICATIONS: ....

DID THE MEDICATION HELP? ....

PHYSICAL ACTIVITY

ACTIVITY/ EXERCISE	DURATION	SETS	REPS	CAL	NOTES

FATIGUE

1 2 3 4 5 6 7 8 9 10

DEPRESSION / ANXIETY

1 2 3 4 5 6 7 8 9 10

MOOD

☆ ☆ ☆ ☆ ☆

TODAY'S DIET

WATER INTAKE

BREAKFAST TIME : ....

....

....

....

CAL : .... CARBS: .... PROTEIN .... FAT ....

LUNCH TIME : ....

....

....

....

....

CAL : .... CARBS: .... PROTEIN .... FAT ....

DINNER TIME : ....

....

....

....

....

CAL : .... CARBS: .... PROTEIN .... FAT ....

SNACKS TIME: ....

....

....

....

....

CAL : .... CARBS: .... PROTEIN .... FAT ....

REACTION TO FOODS

MEAL : ....

FOOD : ....

SYMPTOMS

....

....

....

....

....

HOW MY APPETITE AFFECTED ?

1 2 3 4 5 6 7 8 9 10

NOT AFFECTED NO APPETITE

HOW IS MY URINATION

1 2 3 4 5 6 7 8 9 10

GOOD WORST

HOW IS MY BOWELS

1 2 3 4 5 6 7 8 9 10

CONSTIPATED LOOSE

EXACERBATING CONDITIONS

CURENT WEATHER

SUNNY OVERCAST

FOGGY

RAINY SNOWY

CURRENT WEATHER AFFECTING ME

1 2 3 4 5 6 7 8 9 10

NONE GREATLY

JOB STRESS LEVEL

1 2 3 4 5 6 7 8 9 10

LOW HIGH

TEMPERATURE

LOW HIGH

FAMILY HOME LIFE STRESS LEVEL

1 2 3 4 5 6 7 8 9 10

LOW HIGH

TOP 3 THINGS I WILL DO TO MY CARE-SELF TODAY

....

....

....

TOP 3 THINGS TO ACCOMPLISH TODAY

....

....

....

TOP 3 HIGHLIGHTS OF MY DAY

....

....

....

NOTES /COMMENTS

....

....

....

....

DATE: .... DAY: ....

DAILY QUOTE

"..
...."

	AM	PM
WEIGHT		
TEMPERATURE		
BLOOD PRESSURE		

SUGAR LEVEL

BEFORE BREAKFAST :	AFTER BREAKFAST:
BEFORE LUNCH :	AFTER LUNCH :
BEFORE DINNER :	AFTER DINNER :
BEDTIME :	

SLEEP LAST NIGHT

☐ /HOURS

☐ ☺ ☐ ☹ ☐

NAPS TODAY

☐ /TOTAL HOURS ☐ /HOW MANY

DRUGS/VITAMINS /HERBS/MEDICATIONS	REASON	DOSAGE	TIME			REACTION

SYMPTOM NOTES

RECURRING SYMPTOMS	
NEW SYMPTOMS	

PAIN SITE IDENTIFICATION

MARK PAINFUL AREAS OF THE BODY

OVERALL MORNING PAIN LEVEL

1 2 3 4 5 6 7 8 9 10

LOW HIGH

OVERALL EVENING PAIN LEVEL

1 2 3 4 5 6 7 8 9 10

LOW HIGH

OVERALL AFTERNOON PAIN LEVEL

1 2 3 4 5 6 7 8 9 10

LOW HIGH

SUSPECTED TRIGGERS

....
....

MEDICATIONS: ....

DID THE MEDICATION HELP? ....

PHYSICAL ACTIVITY

ACTIVITY/ EXERCISE	DURATION	SETS	REPS	CAL	NOTES

FATIGUE

1 2 3 4 5 6 7 8 9 10

DEPRESSION / ANXIETY

1 2 3 4 5 6 7 8 9 10

MOOD

☆☆☆☆☆

TODAY'S DIET

WATER INTAKE

BREAKFAST

TIME : ....

CAL : .... CARBS: .... PROTEIN .... FAT ....

LUNCH

TIME : ....

CAL : .... CARBS: .... PROTEIN .... FAT ....

DINNER

TIME : ....

CAL : .... CARBS: .... PROTEIN .... FAT ....

SNACKS

TIME: ....

CAL : .... CARBS: .... PROTEIN .... FAT ....

REACTION TO FOODS

MEAL : ....

FOOD : ....

SYMPTOMS

HOW MY APPETITE AFFECTED ?

1 2 3 4 5 6 7 8 9 10

NOT AFFECTED — NO APPETITE

HOW IS MY URINATION

1 2 3 4 5 6 7 8 9 10

GOOD — WORST

HOW IS MY BOWELS

1 2 3 4 5 6 7 8 9 10

CONSTIPATED — LOOSE

EXACERBATING CONDITIONS

CURENT WEATHER

SUNNY OVERCAST FOGGY RAINY SNOWY

CURRENT WEATHER AFFECTING ME

1 2 3 4 5 6 7 8 9 10

NONE — GREATLY

JOB STRESS LEVEL

1 2 3 4 5 6 7 8 9 10

LOW — HIGH

TEMPERATURE

LOW — HIGH

FAMILY HOME LIFE STRESS LEVEL

1 2 3 4 5 6 7 8 9 10

LOW — HIGH

TOP 3 THINGS I WILL DO TO MY CARE-SELF TODAY

TOP 3 THINGS TO ACCOMPLISH TODAY

TOP 3 HIGHLIGHTS OF MY DAY

NOTES /COMMENTS

DATE: .... DAY: ....

DAILY QUOTE

"..
...."

	AM	PM
WEIGHT		
TEMPERATURE		
BLOOD PRESSURE		

SUGAR LEVEL

BEFORE BREAKFAST :	AFTER BREAKFAST:
BEFORE LUNCH :	AFTER LUNCH :
BEFORE DINNER :	AFTER DINNER :

BEDTIME :

SLEEP LAST NIGHT

/HOURS

NAPS TODAY

/TOTAL HOURS /HOW MANY

DRUGS/VITAMINS /HERBS/MEDICATIONS	REASON	DOSAGE	TIME			REACTION

SYMPTOM NOTES

RECURRING SYMPTOMS	
NEW SYMPTOMS	

PAIN SITE IDENTIFICATION

MARK PAINFUL AREAS OF THE BODY

OVERALL MORNING PAIN LEVEL

1 2 3 4 5 6 7 8 9 10

LOW HIGH

OVERALL AFTERNOON PAIN LEVEL

1 2 3 4 5 6 7 8 9 10

LOW HIGH

OVERALL EVENING PAIN LEVEL

1 2 3 4 5 6 7 8 9 10

LOW HIGH

SUSPECTED TRIGGERS

....
....

MEDICATIONS: ....

DID THE MEDICATION HELP? ....

PHYSICAL ACTIVITY

ACTIVITY/ EXERCISE	DURATION	SETS	REPS	CAL	NOTES

FATIGUE

1 2 3 4 5 6 7 8 9 10

DEPRESSION / ANXIETY

1 2 3 4 5 6 7 8 9 10

MOOD

☆☆☆☆☆

TODAY'S DIET

WATER INTAKE

BREAKFAST TIME :

CAL : CARBS: PROTEIN FAT

LUNCH TIME :

CAL : CARBS: PROTEIN FAT

DINNER TIME :

CAL : CARBS: PROTEIN FAT

SNACKS TIME:

CAL : CARBS: PROTEIN FAT

REACTION TO FOODS

MEAL :

FOOD :

SYMPTOMS

HOW MY APPETITE AFFECTED ?

1 2 3 4 5 6 7 8 9 10

NOT AFFECTED NO APPETITE

HOW IS MY URINATION

1 2 3 4 5 6 7 8 9 10

GOOD WORST

HOW IS MY BOWELS

1 2 3 4 5 6 7 8 9 10

CONSTIPATED LOOSE

EXACERBATING CONDITIONS

CURENT WEATHER

SUNNY OVERCAST

FOGGY

RAINY SNOWY

CURRENT WEATHER AFFECTING ME

1 2 3 4 5 6 7 8 9 10

NONE GREATLY

JOB STRESS LEVEL

1 2 3 4 5 6 7 8 9 10

LOW HIGH

TEMPERATURE

LOW HIGH

FAMILY HOME LIFE STRESS LEVEL

1 2 3 4 5 6 7 8 9 10

LOW HIGH

TOP 3 THINGS I WILL DO TO MY CARE-SELF TODAY

TOP 3 THINGS TO ACCOMPLISH TODAY

TOP 3 HIGHLIGHTS OF MY DAY

NOTES /COMMENTS

DATE: .... DAY: ....

DAILY QUOTE

"..
...."

	AM	PM
WEIGHT		
TEMPERATURE		
BLOOD PRESSURE		

SUGAR LEVEL

BEFORE BREAKFAST :	AFTER BREAKFAST:
BEFORE LUNCH :	AFTER LUNCH :
BEFORE DINNER :	AFTER DINNER :
BEDTIME :	

SLEEP LAST NIGHT

☐ /HOURS

☐ ☺ ☐ ☹ ☐

NAPS TODAY

☐ /TOTAL HOURS ☐ /HOW MANY

DRUGS/VITAMINS /HERBS/MEDICATIONS	REASON	DOSAGE	TIME			REACTION

SYMPTOM NOTES

RECURRING SYMPTOMS	
NEW SYMPTOMS	

PAIN SITE IDENTIFICATION

MARK PAINFUL AREAS OF THE BODY

OVERALL MORNING PAIN LEVEL

1 2 3 4 5 6 7 8 9 10

LOW HIGH

OVERALL AFTERNOON PAIN LEVEL

1 2 3 4 5 6 7 8 9 10

LOW HIGH

OVERALL EVENING PAIN LEVEL

1 2 3 4 5 6 7 8 9 10

LOW HIGH

SUSPECTED TRIGGERS

....
....

MEDICATIONS: ....

DID THE MEDICATION HELP? ....

PHYSICAL ACTIVITY

ACTIVITY/ EXERCISE	DURATION	SETS	REPS	CAL	NOTES

FATIGUE

1 2 3 4 5 6 7 8 9 10

DEPRESSION / ANXIETY

1 2 3 4 5 6 7 8 9 10

MOOD

☆☆☆☆☆

TODAY'S DIET

WATER INTAKE

BREAKFAST TIME : ....

....

CAL : .... CARBS: .... PROTEIN .... FAT ....

LUNCH TIME : ....

....

CAL : .... CARBS: .... PROTEIN .... FAT ....

DINNER TIME : ....

....

CAL : .... CARBS: .... PROTEIN .... FAT ....

SNACKS TIME: ....

....

CAL : .... CARBS: .... PROTEIN .... FAT ....

REACTION TO FOODS

MEAL : ....

FOOD : ....

SYMPTOMS

....

HOW MY APPETITE AFFECTED ?

1 2 3 4 5 6 7 8 9 10

NOT AFFECTED NO APPETITE

HOW IS MY URINATION

1 2 3 4 5 6 7 8 9 10

GOOD WORST

HOW IS MY BOWELS

1 2 3 4 5 6 7 8 9 10

CONSTIPATED LOOSE

EXACERBATING CONDITIONS

CURENT WEATHER

SUNNY OVERCAST

FOGGY

RAINY SNOWY

CURRENT WEATHER AFFECTING ME

1 2 3 4 5 6 7 8 9 10

NONE GREATLY

JOB STRESS LEVEL

1 2 3 4 5 6 7 8 9 10

LOW HIGH

TEMPERATURE

LOW HIGH

FAMILY HOME LIFE STRESS LEVEL

1 2 3 4 5 6 7 8 9 10

LOW HIGH

TOP 3 THINGS I WILL DO TO MY CARE-SELF TODAY

....

TOP 3 THINGS TO ACCOMPLISH TODAY

....

TOP 3 HIGHLIGHTS OF MY DAY

....

NOTES /COMMENTS

....

DATE: .... DAY: ....

DAILY QUOTE

....
....

	AM	PM
WEIGHT		
TEMPERATURE		
BLOOD PRESSURE		

SUGAR LEVEL

BEFORE BREAKFAST :	AFTER BREAKFAST:
BEFORE LUNCH :	AFTER LUNCH :
BEFORE DINNER :	AFTER DINNER :

BEDTIME :

SLEEP LAST NIGHT

☐ /HOURS

☐ ☺ ☐ ☹ ☐

NAPS TODAY

☐ /TOTAL HOURS ☐ /HOW MANY

DRUGS/VITAMINS /HERBS/MEDICATIONS	REASON	DOSAGE	TIME			REACTION

SYMPTOM NOTES

RECURRING SYMPTOMS	
NEW SYMPTOMS	

PAIN SITE IDENTIFICATION

MARK PAINFUL AREAS OF THE BODY

OVERALL MORNING PAIN LEVEL

1 2 3 4 5 6 7 8 9 10

LOW HIGH

OVERALL AFTERNOON PAIN LEVEL

1 2 3 4 5 6 7 8 9 10

LOW HIGH

OVERALL EVENING PAIN LEVEL

1 2 3 4 5 6 7 8 9 10

LOW HIGH

SUSPECTED TRIGGERS

....
....

MEDICATIONS: ....

DID THE MEDICATION HELP? ....

PHYSICAL ACTIVITY

ACTIVITY/ EXERCISE	DURATION	SETS	REPS	CAL	NOTES

FATIGUE

1 2 3 4 5 6 7 8 9 10

DEPRESSION / ANXIETY

1 2 3 4 5 6 7 8 9 10

MOOD

☆ ☆ ☆ ☆ ☆

TODAY'S DIET

WATER INTAKE

BREAKFAST TIME : ....

CAL : .... CARBS: .... PROTEIN .... FAT ....

LUNCH TIME : ....

CAL : .... CARBS: .... PROTEIN .... FAT ....

DINNER TIME : ....

CAL : .... CARBS: .... PROTEIN .... FAT ....

SNACKS TIME: ....

CAL : .... CARBS: .... PROTEIN .... FAT ....

REACTION TO FOODS

MEAL : ....

FOOD : ....

SYMPTOMS

HOW MY APPETITE AFFECTED ?

1 2 3 4 5 6 7 8 9 10

NOT AFFECTED NO APPETITE

HOW IS MY URINATION

1 2 3 4 5 6 7 8 9 10

GOOD WORST

HOW IS MY BOWELS

1 2 3 4 5 6 7 8 9 10

CONSTIPATED LOOSE

EXACERBATING CONDITIONS

CURENT WEATHER

SUNNY OVERCAST

FOGGY

RAINY SNOWY

CURRENT WEATHER AFFECTING ME

1 2 3 4 5 6 7 8 9 10

NONE GREATLY

JOB STRESS LEVEL

1 2 3 4 5 6 7 8 9 10

LOW HIGH

TEMPERATURE

LOW HIGH

FAMILY HOME LIFE STRESS LEVEL

1 2 3 4 5 6 7 8 9 10

LOW HIGH

TOP 3 THINGS I WILL DO TO MY CARE-SELF TODAY

TOP 3 THINGS TO ACCOMPLISH TODAY

TOP 3 HIGHLIGHTS OF MY DAY

NOTES /COMMENTS

DATE: .... DAY: ....

DAILY QUOTE

"..
...."

	AM	PM
WEIGHT		
TEMPERATURE		
BLOOD PRESSURE		

SUGAR LEVEL

BEFORE BREAKFAST :	AFTER BREAKFAST:
BEFORE LUNCH :	AFTER LUNCH :
BEFORE DINNER :	AFTER DINNER :

BEDTIME :

SLEEP LAST NIGHT

☐ /HOURS

☐ ☺ ☐ ☹ ☐

NAPS TODAY

☐ /TOTAL HOURS ☐ /HOW MANY

DRUGS/VITAMINS /HERBS/MEDICATIONS	REASON	DOSAGE	TIME			REACTION

SYMPTOM NOTES

RECURRING SYMPTOMS	
NEW SYMPTOMS	

PAIN SITE IDENTIFICATION

MARK PAINFUL AREAS OF THE BODY

OVERALL MORNING PAIN LEVEL

1 2 3 4 5 6 7 8 9 10

LOW HIGH

OVERALL AFTERNOON PAIN LEVEL

1 2 3 4 5 6 7 8 9 10

LOW HIGH

OVERALL EVENING PAIN LEVEL

1 2 3 4 5 6 7 8 9 10

LOW HIGH

SUSPECTED TRIGGERS

....
....

MEDICATIONS: ....

DID THE MEDICATION HELP? ....

PHYSICAL ACTIVITY

ACTIVITY/ EXERCISE	DURATION	SETS	REPS	CAL	NOTES

FATIGUE

1 2 3 4 5 6 7 8 9 10

DEPRESSION / ANXIETY

1 2 3 4 5 6 7 8 9 10

MOOD

☆☆☆☆☆

TODAY'S DIET

WATER INTAKE

BREAKFAST TIME : ....

CAL : .... CARBS: .... PROTEIN .... FAT ....

LUNCH TIME : ....

CAL : .... CARBS: .... PROTEIN .... FAT ....

DINNER TIME : ....

CAL : .... CARBS: .... PROTEIN .... FAT ....

SNACKS TIME: ....

CAL : .... CARBS: .... PROTEIN .... FAT ....

REACTION TO FOODS

MEAL : ....

FOOD : ....

SYMPTOMS

HOW MY APPETITE AFFECTED ?

1 2 3 4 5 6 7 8 9 10

NOT AFFECTED NO APPETITE

HOW IS MY URINATION

1 2 3 4 5 6 7 8 9 10

GOOD WORST

HOW IS MY BOWELS

1 2 3 4 5 6 7 8 9 10

CONSTIPATED LOOSE

EXACERBATING CONDITIONS

CURENT WEATHER

SUNNY OVERCAST FOGGY RAINY SNOWY

CURRENT WEATHER AFFECTING ME

1 2 3 4 5 6 7 8 9 10

NONE GREATLY

JOB STRESS LEVEL

1 2 3 4 5 6 7 8 9 10

LOW HIGH

TEMPERATURE

LOW HIGH

FAMILY HOME LIFE STRESS LEVEL

1 2 3 4 5 6 7 8 9 10

LOW HIGH

TOP 3 THINGS I WILL DO TO MY CARE-SELF TODAY

TOP 3 THINGS TO ACCOMPLISH TODAY

TOP 3 HIGHLIGHTS OF MY DAY

NOTES /COMMENTS

DATE: .... DAY: ....

DAILY QUOTE

" ....
....
"

	AM	PM
WEIGHT		
TEMPERATURE		
BLOOD PRESSURE		

SUGAR LEVEL

BEFORE BREAKFAST :	AFTER BREAKFAST:
BEFORE LUNCH :	AFTER LUNCH :
BEFORE DINNER :	AFTER DINNER :

BEDTIME :

SLEEP LAST NIGHT

☐ /HOURS

☐ ☺ ☐ ☹ ☐

NAPS TODAY

☐ /TOTAL HOURS ☐ /HOW MANY

DRUGS/VITAMINS /HERBS/MEDICATIONS	REASON	DOSAGE	TIME			REACTION

SYMPTOM NOTES

RECURRING SYMPTOMS	
NEW SYMPTOMS	

PAIN SITE IDENTIFICATION

MARK PAINFUL AREAS OF THE BODY

OVERALL MORNING PAIN LEVEL

1 2 3 4 5 6 7 8 9 10

LOW HIGH

OVERALL AFTERNOON PAIN LEVEL

1 2 3 4 5 6 7 8 9 10

LOW HIGH

OVERALL EVENING PAIN LEVEL

1 2 3 4 5 6 7 8 9 10

LOW HIGH

SUSPECTED TRIGGERS

....
....

MEDICATIONS: ....

DID THE MEDICATION HELP? ....

PHYSICAL ACTIVITY

ACTIVITY/ EXERCISE	DURATION	SETS	REPS	CAL	NOTES

FATIGUE

1 2 3 4 5 6 7 8 9 10

DEPRESSION / ANXIETY

1 2 3 4 5 6 7 8 9 10

MOOD

☆☆☆☆☆

TODAY'S DIET

WATER INTAKE

BREAKFAST TIME : ....

CAL : .... CARBS: .... PROTEIN .... FAT ....

LUNCH TIME : ....

CAL : .... CARBS: .... PROTEIN .... FAT ....

DINNER TIME : ....

CAL : .... CARBS: .... PROTEIN .... FAT ....

SNACKS TIME: ....

CAL : .... CARBS: .... PROTEIN .... FAT ....

REACTION TO FOODS

MEAL : ....

FOOD : ....

SYMPTOMS

HOW MY APPETITE AFFECTED ?

1 2 3 4 5 6 7 8 9 10

NOT AFFECTED NO APPETITE

HOW IS MY URINATION

1 2 3 4 5 6 7 8 9 10

GOOD WORST

HOW IS MY BOWELS

1 2 3 4 5 6 7 8 9 10

CONSTIPATED LOOSE

EXACERBATING CONDITIONS

CURENT WEATHER

SUNNY OVERCAST

FOGGY

RAINY SNOWY

CURRENT WEATHER AFFECTING ME

1 2 3 4 5 6 7 8 9 10

NONE GREATLY

JOB STRESS LEVEL

1 2 3 4 5 6 7 8 9 10

LOW HIGH

TEMPERATURE

LOW HIGH

FAMILY HOME LIFE STRESS LEVEL

1 2 3 4 5 6 7 8 9 10

LOW HIGH

TOP 3 THINGS I WILL DO TO MY CARE-SELF TODAY

....

TOP 3 THINGS TO ACCOMPLISH TODAY

....

TOP 3 HIGHLIGHTS OF MY DAY

....

NOTES /COMMENTS

....

DATE: .... DAY: ....

DAILY QUOTE

"..
...."

	AM	PM
WEIGHT		
TEMPERATURE		
BLOOD PRESSURE		

SUGAR LEVEL

BEFORE BREAKFAST :	AFTER BREAKFAST:
BEFORE LUNCH :	AFTER LUNCH :
BEFORE DINNER :	AFTER DINNER :
BEDTIME :	

SLEEP LAST NIGHT

☐ /HOURS

☐ ☺ ☐ ☹ ☐ 😫

NAPS TODAY

☐ /TOTAL HOURS ☐ /HOW MANY

DRUGS/VITAMINS /HERBS/MEDICATIONS	REASON	DOSAGE	TIME			REACTION

SYMPTOM NOTES

RECURRING SYMPTOMS	
NEW SYMPTOMS	

PAIN SITE IDENTIFICATION

MARK PAINFUL AREAS OF THE BODY

OVERALL MORNING PAIN LEVEL

1 2 3 4 5 6 7 8 9 10

LOW HIGH

OVERALL AFTERNOON PAIN LEVEL

1 2 3 4 5 6 7 8 9 10

LOW HIGH

OVERALL EVENING PAIN LEVEL

1 2 3 4 5 6 7 8 9 10

LOW HIGH

SUSPECTED TRIGGERS

....
....

MEDICATIONS: ....

DID THE MEDICATION HELP? ....

PHYSICAL ACTIVITY

ACTIVITY/ EXERCISE	DURATION	SETS	REPS	CAL	NOTES

FATIGUE

1 2 3 4 5 6 7 8 9 10

DEPRESSION / ANXIETY

1 2 3 4 5 6 7 8 9 10

MOOD

☆ ☆ ☆ ☆ ☆

TODAY'S DIET

WATER INTAKE

BREAKFAST TIME : ....

....
....
....
....

CAL : .... CARBS: .... PROTEIN .... FAT ....

LUNCH TIME : ....

....
....
....
....

CAL : .... CARBS: .... PROTEIN .... FAT ....

DINNER TIME : ....

....
....
....
....

CAL : .... CARBS: .... PROTEIN .... FAT ....

SNACKS TIME: ....

....
....
....
....

CAL : .... CARBS: .... PROTEIN .... FAT ....

REACTION TO FOODS

MEAL : ....

FOOD : ....

SYMPTOMS

....
....
....
....
....

HOW MY APPETITE AFFECTED ?

1 2 3 4 5 6 7 8 9 10

NOT AFFECTED NO APPETITE

HOW IS MY URINATION

1 2 3 4 5 6 7 8 9 10

GOOD WORST

HOW IS MY BOWELS

1 2 3 4 5 6 7 8 9 10

CONSTIPATED LOOSE

EXACERBATING CONDITIONS

CURENT WEATHER

SUNNY OVERCAST

FOGGY

RAINY SNOWY

CURRENT WEATHER AFFECTING ME

1 2 3 4 5 6 7 8 9 10

NONE GREATLY

JOB STRESS LEVEL

1 2 3 4 5 6 7 8 9 10

LOW HIGH

TEMPERATURE

LOW HIGH

FAMILY HOME LIFE STRESS LEVEL

1 2 3 4 5 6 7 8 9 10

LOW HIGH

TOP 3 THINGS I WILL DO TO MY CARE-SELF TODAY

....
....
....

TOP 3 THINGS TO ACCOMPLISH TODAY

....
....
....

TOP 3 HIGHLIGHTS OF MY DAY

....
....
....

NOTES /COMMENTS

....
....
....
....

DATE: .... DAY: ....

DAILY QUOTE

"..
...."

	AM	PM
WEIGHT		
TEMPERATURE		
BLOOD PRESSURE		

SUGAR LEVEL

BEFORE BREAKFAST :	AFTER BREAKFAST:
BEFORE LUNCH :	AFTER LUNCH :
BEFORE DINNER :	AFTER DINNER :
BEDTIME :	

SLEEP LAST NIGHT

☐ /HOURS

☐ ☺ ☐ ☹ ☐

NAPS TODAY

☐ /TOTAL HOURS ☐ /HOW MANY

DRUGS/VITAMINS /HERBS/MEDICATIONS	REASON	DOSAGE	TIME			REACTION

SYMPTOM NOTES

RECURRING SYMPTOMS	
NEW SYMPTOMS	

PAIN SITE IDENTIFICATION

MARK PAINFUL AREAS OF THE BODY

OVERALL MORNING PAIN LEVEL

1 2 3 4 5 6 7 8 9 10

LOW HIGH

OVERALL AFTERNOON PAIN LEVEL

1 2 3 4 5 6 7 8 9 10

LOW HIGH

OVERALL EVENING PAIN LEVEL

1 2 3 4 5 6 7 8 9 10

LOW HIGH

SUSPECTED TRIGGERS

....
....

MEDICATIONS: ....

DID THE MEDICATION HELP? ....

PHYSICAL ACTIVITY

ACTIVITY/ EXERCISE	DURATION	SETS	REPS	CAL	NOTES

FATIGUE

1 2 3 4 5 6 7 8 9 10

DEPRESSION / ANXIETY

1 2 3 4 5 6 7 8 9 10

MOOD

☆☆☆☆☆

TODAY'S DIET

WATER INTAKE

BREAKFAST TIME : ....

CAL : .... CARBS: .... PROTEIN .... FAT ....

LUNCH TIME : ....

CAL : .... CARBS: .... PROTEIN .... FAT ....

DINNER TIME : ....

CAL : .... CARBS: .... PROTEIN .... FAT ....

SNACKS TIME: ....

CAL : .... CARBS: .... PROTEIN .... FAT ....

REACTION TO FOODS

MEAL : ....

FOOD : ....

SYMPTOMS

HOW MY APPETITE AFFECTED ?

1 2 3 4 5 6 7 8 9 10

NOT AFFECTED NO APPETITE

HOW IS MY URINATION

1 2 3 4 5 6 7 8 9 10

GOOD WORST

HOW IS MY BOWELS

1 2 3 4 5 6 7 8 9 10

CONSTIPATED LOOSE

EXACERBATING CONDITIONS

CURENT WEATHER

SUNNY OVERCAST FOGGY RAINY SNOWY

CURRENT WEATHER AFFECTING ME

1 2 3 4 5 6 7 8 9 10

NONE GREATLY

JOB STRESS LEVEL

1 2 3 4 5 6 7 8 9 10

LOW HIGH

TEMPERATURE

LOW HIGH

FAMILY HOME LIFE STRESS LEVEL

1 2 3 4 5 6 7 8 9 10

LOW HIGH

TOP 3 THINGS I WILL DO TO MY CARE-SELF TODAY

TOP 3 THINGS TO ACCOMPLISH TODAY

TOP 3 HIGHLIGHTS OF MY DAY

NOTES /COMMENTS

DATE: .... DAY: ....

DAILY QUOTE

"..
...."

	AM	PM
WEIGHT		
TEMPERATURE		
BLOOD PRESSURE		

SUGAR LEVEL

BEFORE BREAKFAST :	AFTER BREAKFAST:
BEFORE LUNCH :	AFTER LUNCH :
BEFORE DINNER :	AFTER DINNER :

BEDTIME :

SLEEP LAST NIGHT

☐ /HOURS

☐ ☺ ☐ ☹ ☐ 😫

NAPS TODAY

☐ /TOTAL HOURS ☐ /HOW MANY

DRUGS/VITAMINS /HERBS/MEDICATIONS	REASON	DOSAGE	TIME				REACTION

SYMPTOM NOTES

RECURRING SYMPTOMS	
NEW SYMPTOMS	

PAIN SITE IDENTIFICATION

MARK PAINFUL AREAS OF THE BODY

OVERALL MORNING PAIN LEVEL
1 2 3 4 5 6 7 8 9 10
LOW HIGH

OVERALL AFTERNOON PAIN LEVEL
1 2 3 4 5 6 7 8 9 10
LOW HIGH

OVERALL EVENING PAIN LEVEL
1 2 3 4 5 6 7 8 9 10
LOW HIGH

SUSPECTED TRIGGERS

....
....

MEDICATIONS: ....

DID THE MEDICATION HELP? ....

PHYSICAL ACTIVITY

ACTIVITY/ EXERCISE	DURATION	SETS	REPS	CAL	NOTES

FATIGUE
1 2 3 4 5 6 7 8 9 10

DEPRESSION / ANXIETY
1 2 3 4 5 6 7 8 9 10

MOOD
☆☆☆☆☆

TODAY'S DIET

WATER INTAKE

BREAKFAST TIME : ....

CAL : .... CARBS: .... PROTEIN .... FAT ....

LUNCH TIME : ....

CAL : .... CARBS: .... PROTEIN .... FAT ....

DINNER TIME : ....

CAL : .... CARBS: .... PROTEIN .... FAT ....

SNACKS TIME: ....

CAL : .... CARBS: .... PROTEIN .... FAT ....

REACTION TO FOODS

MEAL : ....

FOOD : ....

SYMPTOMS

HOW MY APPETITE AFFECTED ?
1 2 3 4 5 6 7 8 9 10
NOT AFFECTED NO APPETITE

HOW IS MY URINATION
1 2 3 4 5 6 7 8 9 10
GOOD WORST

HOW IS MY BOWELS
1 2 3 4 5 6 7 8 9 10
CONSTIPATED LOOSE

EXACERBATING CONDITIONS

CURENT WEATHER
SUNNY OVERCAST
FOGGY
RAINY SNOWY

CURRENT WEATHER AFFECTING ME
1 2 3 4 5 6 7 8 9 10
NONE GREATLY

JOB STRESS LEVEL
1 2 3 4 5 6 7 8 9 10
LOW HIGH

TEMPERATURE
LOW HIGH

FAMILY HOME LIFE STRESS LEVEL
1 2 3 4 5 6 7 8 9 10
LOW HIGH

TOP 3 THINGS I WILL DO TO MY CARE-SELF TODAY

....

TOP 3 THINGS TO ACCOMPLISH TODAY

....

TOP 3 HIGHLIGHTS OF MY DAY

....

NOTES /COMMENTS

....

DATE: .... DAY: ....

DAILY QUOTE

"..
...."

	AM	PM
WEIGHT		
TEMPERATURE		
BLOOD PRESSURE		

SUGAR LEVEL

BEFORE BREAKFAST :	AFTER BREAKFAST:
BEFORE LUNCH :	AFTER LUNCH :
BEFORE DINNER :	AFTER DINNER :

BEDTIME :

SLEEP LAST NIGHT

☐ /HOURS

☐ ☺ ☐ ☹ ☐ 😫

NAPS TODAY

☐ /TOTAL HOURS ☐ /HOW MANY

DRUGS/VITAMINS /HERBS/MEDICATIONS	REASON	DOSAGE	TIME			REACTION

SYMPTOM NOTES

RECURRING SYMPTOMS	
NEW SYMPTOMS	

PAIN SITE IDENTIFICATION

MARK PAINFUL AREAS OF THE BODY

OVERALL MORNING PAIN LEVEL

1 2 3 4 5 6 7 8 9 10

LOW HIGH

OVERALL AFTERNOON PAIN LEVEL

1 2 3 4 5 6 7 8 9 10

LOW HIGH

OVERALL EVENING PAIN LEVEL

1 2 3 4 5 6 7 8 9 10

LOW HIGH

SUSPECTED TRIGGERS

....
....

MEDICATIONS: ....

DID THE MEDICATION HELP? ....

PHYSICAL ACTIVITY

ACTIVITY/ EXERCISE	DURATION	SETS	REPS	CAL	NOTES

FATIGUE

1 2 3 4 5 6 7 8 9 10

DEPRESSION / ANXIETY

1 2 3 4 5 6 7 8 9 10

MOOD

☆☆☆☆☆

TODAY'S DIET

WATER INTAKE

BREAKFAST TIME : ....

....
....
....

CAL : .... CARBS: .... PROTEIN .... FAT ....

LUNCH TIME : ....

....
....
....

CAL : .... CARBS: .... PROTEIN .... FAT ....

DINNER TIME : ....

....
....
....

CAL : .... CARBS: .... PROTEIN .... FAT ....

SNACKS TIME: ....

....
....
....

CAL : .... CARBS: .... PROTEIN .... FAT ....

REACTION TO FOODS

MEAL : ....

FOOD : ....

SYMPTOMS

....
....
....
....
....

HOW MY APPETITE AFFECTED ?

1 2 3 4 5 6 7 8 9 10

NOT AFFECTED NO APPETITE

HOW IS MY URINATION

1 2 3 4 5 6 7 8 9 10

GOOD WORST

HOW IS MY BOWELS

1 2 3 4 5 6 7 8 9 10

CONSTIPATED LOOSE

EXACERBATING CONDITIONS

CURENT WEATHER

SUNNY OVERCAST

FOGGY

RAINY SNOWY

CURRENT WEATHER AFFECTING ME

1 2 3 4 5 6 7 8 9 10

NONE GREATLY

JOB STRESS LEVEL

1 2 3 4 5 6 7 8 9 10

LOW HIGH

TEMPERATURE

LOW HIGH

FAMILY HOME LIFE STRESS LEVEL

1 2 3 4 5 6 7 8 9 10

LOW HIGH

TOP 3 THINGS I WILL DO TO MY CARE-SELF TODAY

....
....
....

TOP 3 THINGS TO ACCOMPLISH TODAY

....
....
....

TOP 3 HIGHLIGHTS OF MY DAY

....
....
....

NOTES /COMMENTS

....
....
....
....

DATE: .... DAY: ....

DAILY QUOTE

"..
...."

	AM	PM
WEIGHT		
TEMPERATURE		
BLOOD PRESSURE		

SUGAR LEVEL

BEFORE BREAKFAST :	AFTER BREAKFAST:
BEFORE LUNCH :	AFTER LUNCH :
BEFORE DINNER :	AFTER DINNER :

BEDTIME :

SLEEP LAST NIGHT

☐ /HOURS

☐ ☺ ☐ ☹ ☐

NAPS TODAY

☐ /TOTAL HOURS ☐ /HOW MANY

DRUGS/VITAMINS /HERBS/MEDICATIONS	REASON	DOSAGE	TIME			REACTION

SYMPTOM NOTES

RECURRING SYMPTOMS	
NEW SYMPTOMS	

PAIN SITE IDENTIFICATION

MARK PAINFUL AREAS OF THE BODY

OVERALL MORNING PAIN LEVEL

1 2 3 4 5 6 7 8 9 10

LOW HIGH

OVERALL AFTERNOON PAIN LEVEL

1 2 3 4 5 6 7 8 9 10

LOW HIGH

OVERALL EVENING PAIN LEVEL

1 2 3 4 5 6 7 8 9 10

LOW HIGH

SUSPECTED TRIGGERS

....
....

MEDICATIONS: ....

DID THE MEDICATION HELP? ....

PHYSICAL ACTIVITY

ACTIVITY/ EXERCISE	DURATION	SETS	REPS	CAL	NOTES

FATIGUE

1 2 3 4 5 6 7 8 9 10

DEPRESSION / ANXIETY

1 2 3 4 5 6 7 8 9 10

MOOD

☆☆☆☆☆

TODAY'S DIET

WATER INTAKE

BREAKFAST TIME : ....

....

....

....

CAL : .... CARBS: .... PROTEIN .... FAT ....

LUNCH TIME : ....

....

....

....

CAL : .... CARBS: .... PROTEIN .... FAT ....

DINNER TIME : ....

....

....

....

CAL : .... CARBS: .... PROTEIN .... FAT ....

SNACKS TIME: ....

....

....

....

CAL : .... CARBS: .... PROTEIN .... FAT ....

REACTION TO FOODS

MEAL : ....

FOOD : ....

SYMPTOMS

....

....

....

....

....

HOW MY APPETITE AFFECTED ?

1 2 3 4 5 6 7 8 9 10

NOT AFFECTED NO APPETITE

HOW IS MY URINATION

1 2 3 4 5 6 7 8 9 10

GOOD WORST

HOW IS MY BOWELS

1 2 3 4 5 6 7 8 9 10

CONSTIPATED LOOSE

EXACERBATING CONDITIONS

CURENT WEATHER

SUNNY OVERCAST

FOGGY

RAINY SNOWY

CURRENT WEATHER AFFECTING ME

1 2 3 4 5 6 7 8 9 10

NONE GREATLY

JOB STRESS LEVEL

1 2 3 4 5 6 7 8 9 10

LOW HIGH

TEMPERATURE

LOW HIGH

FAMILY HOME LIFE STRESS LEVEL

1 2 3 4 5 6 7 8 9 10

LOW HIGH

TOP 3 THINGS I WILL DO TO MY CARE-SELF TODAY

....

....

....

TOP 3 THINGS TO ACCOMPLISH TODAY

....

....

....

TOP 3 HIGHLIGHTS OF MY DAY

....

....

....

NOTES /COMMENTS

....

....

....

....

DATE: .... DAY: ....

DAILY QUOTE

"...
...."

	AM	PM
WEIGHT		
TEMPERATURE		
BLOOD PRESSURE		

SUGAR LEVEL

BEFORE BREAKFAST :	AFTER BREAKFAST:
BEFORE LUNCH :	AFTER LUNCH :
BEFORE DINNER :	AFTER DINNER :

BEDTIME :

SLEEP LAST NIGHT

☐ /HOURS

☐ ☺ ☐ ☹ ☐

NAPS TODAY

☐ /TOTAL HOURS ☐ /HOW MANY

DRUGS/VITAMINS /HERBS/MEDICATIONS	REASON	DOSAGE	TIME			REACTION

SYMPTOM NOTES	
RECURRING SYMPTOMS	
NEW SYMPTOMS	

PAIN SITE IDENTIFICATION

MARK PAINFUL AREAS OF THE BODY

OVERALL MORNING PAIN LEVEL

1 2 3 4 5 6 7 8 9 10

LOW HIGH

OVERALL AFTERNOON PAIN LEVEL

1 2 3 4 5 6 7 8 9 10

LOW HIGH

OVERALL EVENING PAIN LEVEL

1 2 3 4 5 6 7 8 9 10

LOW HIGH

SUSPECTED TRIGGERS

....
....

MEDICATIONS: ....

DID THE MEDICATION HELP? ....

PHYSICAL ACTIVITY

ACTIVITY/ EXERCISE	DURATION	SETS	REPS	CAL	NOTES

FATIGUE

1 2 3 4 5 6 7 8 9 10

DEPRESSION / ANXIETY

1 2 3 4 5 6 7 8 9 10

MOOD

☆☆☆☆☆

TODAY'S DIET

WATER INTAKE

BREAKFAST TIME : ....

CAL : .... CARBS: .... PROTEIN .... FAT ....

LUNCH TIME : ....

CAL : .... CARBS: .... PROTEIN .... FAT ....

DINNER TIME : ....

CAL : .... CARBS: .... PROTEIN .... FAT ....

SNACKS TIME: ....

CAL : .... CARBS: .... PROTEIN .... FAT ....

REACTION TO FOODS

MEAL : ....

FOOD : ....

SYMPTOMS

....

HOW MY APPETITE AFFECTED ?

1 2 3 4 5 6 7 8 9 10

NOT AFFECTED NO APPETITE

HOW IS MY URINATION

1 2 3 4 5 6 7 8 9 10

GOOD WORST

HOW IS MY BOWELS

1 2 3 4 5 6 7 8 9 10

CONSTIPATED LOOSE

EXACERBATING CONDITIONS

CURENT WEATHER

SUNNY OVERCAST

FOGGY

RAINY SNOWY

CURRENT WEATHER AFFECTING ME

1 2 3 4 5 6 7 8 9 10

NONE GREATLY

JOB STRESS LEVEL

1 2 3 4 5 6 7 8 9 10

LOW HIGH

TEMPERATURE

LOW HIGH

FAMILY HOME LIFE STRESS LEVEL

1 2 3 4 5 6 7 8 9 10

LOW HIGH

TOP 3 THINGS I WILL DO TO MY CARE-SELF TODAY

....

TOP 3 THINGS TO ACCOMPLISH TODAY

....

TOP 3 HIGHLIGHTS OF MY DAY

....

NOTES /COMMENTS

....

DATE: .... DAY: ....

DAILY QUOTE

"..
...."

	AM	PM
WEIGHT		
TEMPERATURE		
BLOOD PRESSURE		

SUGAR LEVEL

BEFORE BREAKFAST :	AFTER BREAKFAST:
BEFORE LUNCH :	AFTER LUNCH :
BEFORE DINNER :	AFTER DINNER :

BEDTIME :

SLEEP LAST NIGHT

☐ /HOURS

☐ ☺ ☐ ☹ ☐

NAPS TODAY

☐ /TOTAL HOURS ☐ /HOW MANY

DRUGS/VITAMINS /HERBS/MEDICATIONS	REASON	DOSAGE	TIME			REACTION

SYMPTOM NOTES

RECURRING SYMPTOMS	
NEW SYMPTOMS	

PAIN SITE IDENTIFICATION

MARK PAINFUL AREAS OF THE BODY

OVERALL MORNING PAIN LEVEL

1 2 3 4 5 6 7 8 9 10

LOW HIGH

OVERALL AFTERNOON PAIN LEVEL

1 2 3 4 5 6 7 8 9 10

LOW HIGH

OVERALL EVENING PAIN LEVEL

1 2 3 4 5 6 7 8 9 10

LOW HIGH

SUSPECTED TRIGGERS

....
....

MEDICATIONS: ....

DID THE MEDICATION HELP? ....

PHYSICAL ACTIVITY

ACTIVITY/ EXERCISE	DURATION	SETS	REPS	CAL	NOTES

FATIGUE

1 2 3 4 5 6 7 8 9 10

DEPRESSION / ANXIETY

1 2 3 4 5 6 7 8 9 10

MOOD

☆☆☆☆☆

TODAY'S DIET

WATER INTAKE

BREAKFAST TIME : ....

....
....
....
....

CAL : .... CARBS: .... PROTEIN .... FAT ....

LUNCH TIME : ....

....
....
....
....

CAL : .... CARBS: .... PROTEIN .... FAT ....

DINNER TIME : ....

....
....
....
....

CAL : .... CARBS: .... PROTEIN .... FAT ....

SNACKS TIME: ....

....
....
....
....

CAL : .... CARBS: .... PROTEIN .... FAT ....

REACTION TO FOODS

MEAL : ....

FOOD : ....

SYMPTOMS

....
....
....
....
....

HOW MY APPETITE AFFECTED ?

1 2 3 4 5 6 7 8 9 10

NOT AFFECTED NO APPETITE

HOW IS MY URINATION

1 2 3 4 5 6 7 8 9 10

GOOD WORST

HOW IS MY BOWELS

1 2 3 4 5 6 7 8 9 10

CONSTIPATED LOOSE

EXACERBATING CONDITIONS

CURENT WEATHER

SUNNY OVERCAST

FOGGY

RAINY SNOWY

CURRENT WEATHER AFFECTING ME

1 2 3 4 5 6 7 8 9 10

NONE GREATLY

JOB STRESS LEVEL

1 2 3 4 5 6 7 8 9 10

LOW HIGH

TEMPERATURE

LOW HIGH

FAMILY HOME LIFE STRESS LEVEL

1 2 3 4 5 6 7 8 9 10

LOW HIGH

TOP 3 THINGS I WILL DO TO MY CARE-SELF TODAY

....
....
....

TOP 3 THINGS TO ACCOMPLISH TODAY

....
....
....

TOP 3 HIGHLIGHTS OF MY DAY

....
....
....

NOTES /COMMENTS

....
....
....
....

DATE: .... DAY: ....

DAILY QUOTE

"..
...."

	AM	PM
WEIGHT		
TEMPERATURE		
BLOOD PRESSURE		

SUGAR LEVEL

BEFORE BREAKFAST :	AFTER BREAKFAST:
BEFORE LUNCH :	AFTER LUNCH :
BEFORE DINNER :	AFTER DINNER :

BEDTIME :

SLEEP LAST NIGHT

☐ /HOURS

☐ ☺ ☐ ☹ ☐ 😫

NAPS TODAY

☐ /TOTAL HOURS ☐ /HOW MANY

DRUGS/VITAMINS /HERBS/MEDICATIONS	REASON	DOSAGE	TIME			REACTION

SYMPTOM NOTES

RECURRING SYMPTOMS	
NEW SYMPTOMS	

PAIN SITE IDENTIFICATION

MARK PAINFUL AREAS OF THE BODY

OVERALL MORNING PAIN LEVEL

1 2 3 4 5 6 7 8 9 10

LOW HIGH

OVERALL EVENING PAIN LEVEL

1 2 3 4 5 6 7 8 9 10

LOW HIGH

OVERALL AFTERNOON PAIN LEVEL

1 2 3 4 5 6 7 8 9 10

LOW HIGH

SUSPECTED TRIGGERS

....
....

MEDICATIONS: ....

DID THE MEDICATION HELP? ....

PHYSICAL ACTIVITY

ACTIVITY/ EXERCISE	DURATION	SETS	REPS	CAL	NOTES

FATIGUE

1 2 3 4 5 6 7 8 9 10

DEPRESSION / ANXIETY

1 2 3 4 5 6 7 8 9 10

MOOD

☆☆☆☆☆

TODAY'S DIET

WATER INTAKE

BREAKFAST TIME : ....

CAL : .... CARBS: .... PROTEIN .... FAT ....

LUNCH TIME : ....

CAL : .... CARBS: .... PROTEIN .... FAT ....

DINNER TIME : ....

CAL : .... CARBS: .... PROTEIN .... FAT ....

SNACKS TIME: ....

CAL : .... CARBS: .... PROTEIN .... FAT ....

REACTION TO FOODS

MEAL : ....

FOOD : ....

SYMPTOMS

HOW MY APPETITE AFFECTED ?
1 2 3 4 5 6 7 8 9 10
NOT AFFECTED NO APPETITE

HOW IS MY URINATION
1 2 3 4 5 6 7 8 9 10
GOOD WORST

HOW IS MY BOWELS
1 2 3 4 5 6 7 8 9 10
CONSTIPATED LOOSE

EXACERBATING CONDITIONS

CURENT WEATHER
SUNNY OVERCAST
FOGGY
RAINY SNOWY

CURRENT WEATHER AFFECTING ME
1 2 3 4 5 6 7 8 9 10
NONE GREATLY

JOB STRESS LEVEL
1 2 3 4 5 6 7 8 9 10
LOW HIGH

TEMPERATURE
LOW HIGH

FAMILY HOME LIFE STRESS LEVEL
1 2 3 4 5 6 7 8 9 10
LOW HIGH

TOP 3 THINGS I WILL DO TO MY CARE-SELF TODAY

TOP 3 THINGS TO ACCOMPLISH TODAY

TOP 3 HIGHLIGHTS OF MY DAY

NOTES /COMMENTS

DATE: .... DAY: ....

DAILY QUOTE

"..
...."

	AM	PM
WEIGHT		
TEMPERATURE		
BLOOD PRESSURE		

SUGAR LEVEL

BEFORE BREAKFAST :	AFTER BREAKFAST:
BEFORE LUNCH :	AFTER LUNCH :
BEFORE DINNER :	AFTER DINNER :

BEDTIME :

SLEEP LAST NIGHT

☐ /HOURS

☐ ☺ ☐ ☹ ☐

NAPS TODAY

☐ /TOTAL HOURS ☐ /HOW MANY

DRUGS/VITAMINS /HERBS/MEDICATIONS	REASON	DOSAGE	TIME			REACTION

SYMPTOM NOTES

RECURRING SYMPTOMS	
NEW SYMPTOMS	

PAIN SITE IDENTIFICATION

MARK PAINFUL AREAS OF THE BODY

OVERALL MORNING PAIN LEVEL

1 2 3 4 5 6 7 8 9 10

LOW HIGH

OVERALL EVENING PAIN LEVEL

1 2 3 4 5 6 7 8 9 10

LOW HIGH

OVERALL AFTERNOON PAIN LEVEL

1 2 3 4 5 6 7 8 9 10

LOW HIGH

SUSPECTED TRIGGERS

....
....

MEDICATIONS: ....

DID THE MEDICATION HELP? ....

PHYSICAL ACTIVITY

ACTIVITY/ EXERCISE	DURATION	SETS	REPS	CAL	NOTES

FATIGUE

1 2 3 4 5 6 7 8 9 10

DEPRESSION / ANXIETY

1 2 3 4 5 6 7 8 9 10

MOOD

☆ ☆ ☆ ☆ ☆

TODAY'S DIET

WATER INTAKE

BREAKFAST TIME :

CAL : CARBS: PROTEIN FAT

LUNCH TIME :

CAL : CARBS: PROTEIN FAT

DINNER TIME :

CAL : CARBS: PROTEIN FAT

SNACKS TIME:

CAL : CARBS: PROTEIN FAT

REACTION TO FOODS

MEAL :

FOOD :

SYMPTOMS

HOW MY APPETITE AFFECTED ?

1 2 3 4 5 6 7 8 9 10

NOT AFFECTED NO APPETITE

HOW IS MY URINATION

1 2 3 4 5 6 7 8 9 10

GOOD WORST

HOW IS MY BOWELS

1 2 3 4 5 6 7 8 9 10

CONSTIPATED LOOSE

EXACERBATING CONDITIONS

CURENT WEATHER

SUNNY OVERCAST

FOGGY

RAINY SNOWY

CURRENT WEATHER AFFECTING ME

1 2 3 4 5 6 7 8 9 10

NONE GREATLY

JOB STRESS LEVEL

1 2 3 4 5 6 7 8 9 10

LOW HIGH

TEMPERATURE

LOW HIGH

FAMILY HOME LIFE STRESS LEVEL

1 2 3 4 5 6 7 8 9 10

LOW HIGH

TOP 3 THINGS I WILL DO TO MY CARE-SELF TODAY

TOP 3 THINGS TO ACCOMPLISH TODAY

TOP 3 HIGHLIGHTS OF MY DAY

NOTES /COMMENTS

DATE: .... DAY: ....

DAILY QUOTE

" ....
.... "

	AM	PM
WEIGHT		
TEMPERATURE		
BLOOD PRESSURE		

SUGAR LEVEL

BEFORE BREAKFAST :	AFTER BREAKFAST:
BEFORE LUNCH :	AFTER LUNCH :
BEFORE DINNER :	AFTER DINNER :

BEDTIME :

SLEEP LAST NIGHT

☐ /HOURS

☐ ☺ ☐ ☹ ☐

NAPS TODAY

☐ /TOTAL HOURS ☐ /HOW MANY

DRUGS/VITAMINS /HERBS/MEDICATIONS	REASON	DOSAGE	TIME			REACTION

SYMPTOM NOTES

RECURRING SYMPTOMS	
NEW SYMPTOMS	

PAIN SITE IDENTIFICATION

MARK PAINFUL AREAS OF THE BODY

OVERALL MORNING PAIN LEVEL

1 2 3 4 5 6 7 8 9 10

LOW HIGH

OVERALL AFTERNOON PAIN LEVEL

1 2 3 4 5 6 7 8 9 10

LOW HIGH

OVERALL EVENING PAIN LEVEL

1 2 3 4 5 6 7 8 9 10

LOW HIGH

SUSPECTED TRIGGERS

....
....

MEDICATIONS: ....

DID THE MEDICATION HELP? ....

PHYSICAL ACTIVITY

ACTIVITY/ EXERCISE	DURATION	SETS	REPS	CAL	NOTES

FATIGUE

1 2 3 4 5 6 7 8 9 10

DEPRESSION / ANXIETY

1 2 3 4 5 6 7 8 9 10

MOOD

☆☆☆☆☆

TODAY'S DIET

WATER INTAKE

BREAKFAST TIME : ....

CAL : .... CARBS: .... PROTEIN .... FAT ....

LUNCH TIME : ....

CAL : .... CARBS: .... PROTEIN .... FAT ....

DINNER TIME : ....

CAL : .... CARBS: .... PROTEIN .... FAT ....

SNACKS TIME: ....

CAL : .... CARBS: .... PROTEIN .... FAT ....

REACTION TO FOODS

MEAL : ....

FOOD : ....

SYMPTOMS

HOW MY APPETITE AFFECTED ?

1 2 3 4 5 6 7 8 9 10

NOT AFFECTED NO APPETITE

HOW IS MY URINATION

1 2 3 4 5 6 7 8 9 10

GOOD WORST

HOW IS MY BOWELS

1 2 3 4 5 6 7 8 9 10

CONSTIPATED LOOSE

EXACERBATING CONDITIONS

CURENT WEATHER

SUNNY OVERCAST FOGGY RAINY SNOWY

CURRENT WEATHER AFFECTING ME

1 2 3 4 5 6 7 8 9 10

NONE GREATLY

JOB STRESS LEVEL

1 2 3 4 5 6 7 8 9 10

LOW HIGH

TEMPERATURE

LOW HIGH

FAMILY HOME LIFE STRESS LEVEL

1 2 3 4 5 6 7 8 9 10

LOW HIGH

TOP 3 THINGS I WILL DO TO MY CARE-SELF TODAY

TOP 3 THINGS TO ACCOMPLISH TODAY

TOP 3 HIGHLIGHTS OF MY DAY

NOTES /COMMENTS

DATE:.................. DAY: ....

DAILY QUOTE

"..
...."

	AM	PM
WEIGHT		
TEMPERATURE		
BLOOD PRESSURE		

SUGAR LEVEL

BEFORE BREAKFAST :	AFTER BREAKFAST:
BEFORE LUNCH :	AFTER LUNCH :
BEFORE DINNER :	AFTER DINNER :

BEDTIME :

SLEEP LAST NIGHT

☐ /HOURS

☐ ☺ ☐ ☹ ☐

NAPS TODAY

☐ /TOTAL HOURS ☐ /HOW MANY

DRUGS/VITAMINS /HERBS/MEDICATIONS	REASON	DOSAGE	TIME			REACTION

SYMPTOM NOTES

RECURRING SYMPTOMS	
NEW SYMPTOMS	

PAIN SITE IDENTIFICATION

MARK PAINFUL AREAS OF THE BODY

OVERALL MORNING PAIN LEVEL

1 2 3 4 5 6 7 8 9 10

LOW HIGH

OVERALL AFTERNOON PAIN LEVEL

1 2 3 4 5 6 7 8 9 10

LOW HIGH

OVERALL EVENING PAIN LEVEL

1 2 3 4 5 6 7 8 9 10

LOW HIGH

SUSPECTED TRIGGERS

....
....

MEDICATIONS: ....

DID THE MEDICATION HELP? ....

PHYSICAL ACTIVITY

ACTIVITY/ EXERCISE	DURATION	SETS	REPS	CAL	NOTES

FATIGUE

1 2 3 4 5 6 7 8 9 10

DEPRESSION / ANXIETY

1 2 3 4 5 6 7 8 9 10

MOOD

☆☆☆☆☆

TODAY'S DIET

WATER INTAKE

BREAKFAST TIME : ....

....

CAL : .... CARBS: .... PROTEIN .... FAT ....

LUNCH TIME : ....

....

CAL : .... CARBS: .... PROTEIN .... FAT ....

DINNER TIME : ....

....

CAL : .... CARBS: .... PROTEIN .... FAT ....

SNACKS TIME: ....

....

CAL : .... CARBS: .... PROTEIN .... FAT ....

REACTION TO FOODS

MEAL : ....

FOOD : ....

SYMPTOMS

....

HOW MY APPETITE AFFECTED ?

1 2 3 4 5 6 7 8 9 10

NOT AFFECTED NO APPETITE

HOW IS MY URINATION

1 2 3 4 5 6 7 8 9 10

GOOD WORST

HOW IS MY BOWELS

1 2 3 4 5 6 7 8 9 10

CONSTIPATED LOOSE

EXACERBATING CONDITIONS

CURENT WEATHER

SUNNY OVERCAST FOGGY RAINY SNOWY

CURRENT WEATHER AFFECTING ME

1 2 3 4 5 6 7 8 9 10

NONE GREATLY

JOB STRESS LEVEL

1 2 3 4 5 6 7 8 9 10

LOW HIGH

TEMPERATURE

LOW HIGH

FAMILY HOME LIFE STRESS LEVEL

1 2 3 4 5 6 7 8 9 10

LOW HIGH

TOP 3 THINGS I WILL DO TO MY CARE-SELF TODAY

....

TOP 3 THINGS TO ACCOMPLISH TODAY

....

TOP 3 HIGHLIGHTS OF MY DAY

....

NOTES /COMMENTS

....

DATE:.................... DAY: ....

DAILY QUOTE

"...
...."

	AM	PM
WEIGHT		
TEMPERATURE		
BLOOD PRESSURE		

SUGAR LEVEL

BEFORE BREAKFAST :	AFTER BREAKFAST:
BEFORE LUNCH :	AFTER LUNCH :
BEFORE DINNER :	AFTER DINNER :

BEDTIME :

SLEEP LAST NIGHT

☐ /HOURS

☐ ☺ ☐ ☹ ☐ 😫

NAPS TODAY

☐ /TOTAL HOURS ☐ /HOW MANY

DRUGS/VITAMINS /HERBS/MEDICATIONS	REASON	DOSAGE	TIME			REACTION

SYMPTOM NOTES

RECURRING SYMPTOMS	
NEW SYMPTOMS	

PAIN SITE IDENTIFICATION

MARK PAINFUL AREAS OF THE BODY

OVERALL MORNING PAIN LEVEL

1 2 3 4 5 6 7 8 9 10

LOW HIGH

OVERALL AFTERNOON PAIN LEVEL

1 2 3 4 5 6 7 8 9 10

LOW HIGH

OVERALL EVENING PAIN LEVEL

1 2 3 4 5 6 7 8 9 10

LOW HIGH

SUSPECTED TRIGGERS

....
....

MEDICATIONS: ....

DID THE MEDICATION HELP? ....

PHYSICAL ACTIVITY

ACTIVITY/ EXERCISE	DURATION	SETS	REPS	CAL	NOTES

FATIGUE

1 2 3 4 5 6 7 8 9 10

DEPRESSION / ANXIETY

1 2 3 4 5 6 7 8 9 10

MOOD

☆☆☆☆☆

TODAY'S DIET

WATER INTAKE

BREAKFAST TIME : ....

CAL : .... CARBS: .... PROTEIN .... FAT ....

LUNCH TIME : ....

CAL : .... CARBS: .... PROTEIN .... FAT ....

DINNER TIME : ....

CAL : .... CARBS: .... PROTEIN .... FAT ....

SNACKS TIME: ....

CAL : .... CARBS: .... PROTEIN .... FAT ....

REACTION TO FOODS

MEAL : ....

FOOD : ....

SYMPTOMS

HOW MY APPETITE AFFECTED ?

1 2 3 4 5 6 7 8 9 10

NOT AFFECTED NO APPETITE

HOW IS MY URINATION

1 2 3 4 5 6 7 8 9 10

GOOD WORST

HOW IS MY BOWELS

1 2 3 4 5 6 7 8 9 10

CONSTIPATED LOOSE

EXACERBATING CONDITIONS

CURENT WEATHER

SUNNY OVERCAST

FOGGY

RAINY SNOWY

CURRENT WEATHER AFFECTING ME

1 2 3 4 5 6 7 8 9 10

NONE GREATLY

JOB STRESS LEVEL

1 2 3 4 5 6 7 8 9 10

LOW HIGH

TEMPERATURE

LOW HIGH

FAMILY HOME LIFE STRESS LEVEL

1 2 3 4 5 6 7 8 9 10

LOW HIGH

TOP 3 THINGS I WILL DO TO MY CARE-SELF TODAY

TOP 3 THINGS TO ACCOMPLISH TODAY

TOP 3 HIGHLIGHTS OF MY DAY

NOTES /COMMENTS

DATE: .... DAY: ....

DAILY QUOTE

" ....
.... "

	AM	PM
WEIGHT		
TEMPERATURE		
BLOOD PRESSURE		

SUGAR LEVEL

BEFORE BREAKFAST :	AFTER BREAKFAST:
BEFORE LUNCH :	AFTER LUNCH :
BEFORE DINNER :	AFTER DINNER :

BEDTIME :

SLEEP LAST NIGHT

☐ /HOURS

☐ ☺ ☐ ☹ ☐ 😫

NAPS TODAY

☐ /TOTAL HOURS ☐ /HOW MANY

DRUGS/VITAMINS /HERBS/MEDICATIONS	REASON	DOSAGE	TIME			REACTION

SYMPTOM NOTES

RECURRING SYMPTOMS	
NEW SYMPTOMS	

PAIN SITE IDENTIFICATION

MARK PAINFUL AREAS OF THE BODY

OVERALL MORNING PAIN LEVEL

1 2 3 4 5 6 7 8 9 10

LOW HIGH

OVERALL AFTERNOON PAIN LEVEL

1 2 3 4 5 6 7 8 9 10

LOW HIGH

OVERALL EVENING PAIN LEVEL

1 2 3 4 5 6 7 8 9 10

LOW HIGH

SUSPECTED TRIGGERS

....
....

MEDICATIONS: ....

DID THE MEDICATION HELP? ....

PHYSICAL ACTIVITY

ACTIVITY/ EXERCISE	DURATION	SETS	REPS	CAL	NOTES

FATIGUE

1 2 3 4 5 6 7 8 9 10

DEPRESSION / ANXIETY

1 2 3 4 5 6 7 8 9 10

MOOD

☆☆☆☆☆

TODAY'S DIET

WATER INTAKE

BREAKFAST TIME : ....

CAL : .... CARBS: .... PROTEIN .... FAT ....

LUNCH TIME : ....

CAL : .... CARBS: .... PROTEIN .... FAT ....

DINNER TIME : ....

CAL : .... CARBS: .... PROTEIN .... FAT ....

SNACKS TIME: ....

CAL : .... CARBS: .... PROTEIN .... FAT ....

REACTION TO FOODS

MEAL : ....

FOOD : ....

SYMPTOMS

HOW MY APPETITE AFFECTED ?

1 2 3 4 5 6 7 8 9 10

NOT AFFECTED NO APPETITE

HOW IS MY URINATION

1 2 3 4 5 6 7 8 9 10

GOOD WORST

HOW IS MY BOWELS

1 2 3 4 5 6 7 8 9 10

CONSTIPATED LOOSE

EXACERBATING CONDITIONS

CURENT WEATHER

SUNNY OVERCAST

FOGGY

RAINY SNOWY

CURRENT WEATHER AFFECTING ME

1 2 3 4 5 6 7 8 9 10

NONE GREATLY

JOB STRESS LEVEL

1 2 3 4 5 6 7 8 9 10

LOW HIGH

TEMPERATURE

LOW HIGH

FAMILY HOME LIFE STRESS LEVEL

1 2 3 4 5 6 7 8 9 10

LOW HIGH

TOP 3 THINGS I WILL DO TO MY CARE-SELF TODAY

TOP 3 THINGS TO ACCOMPLISH TODAY

TOP 3 HIGHLIGHTS OF MY DAY

NOTES /COMMENTS

DATE: .... DAY: ....

DAILY QUOTE

" ....
.... "

	AM	PM
WEIGHT		
TEMPERATURE		
BLOOD PRESSURE		

SUGAR LEVEL

BEFORE BREAKFAST :	AFTER BREAKFAST:
BEFORE LUNCH :	AFTER LUNCH :
BEFORE DINNER :	AFTER DINNER :
BEDTIME :	

SLEEP LAST NIGHT

☐ /HOURS

☐ ☺ ☐ ☹ ☐

NAPS TODAY

☐ /TOTAL HOURS ☐ /HOW MANY

DRUGS/VITAMINS /HERBS/MEDICATIONS	REASON	DOSAGE	TIME			REACTION

SYMPTOM NOTES

RECURRING SYMPTOMS	
NEW SYMPTOMS	

PAIN SITE IDENTIFICATION

MARK PAINFUL AREAS OF THE BODY

OVERALL MORNING PAIN LEVEL

1 2 3 4 5 6 7 8 9 10

LOW HIGH

OVERALL AFTERNOON PAIN LEVEL

1 2 3 4 5 6 7 8 9 10

LOW HIGH

OVERALL EVENING PAIN LEVEL

1 2 3 4 5 6 7 8 9 10

LOW HIGH

SUSPECTED TRIGGERS

....
....

MEDICATIONS: ....

DID THE MEDICATION HELP? ....

PHYSICAL ACTIVITY

ACTIVITY/ EXERCISE	DURATION	SETS	REPS	CAL	NOTES

FATIGUE

1 2 3 4 5 6 7 8 9 10

DEPRESSION / ANXIETY

1 2 3 4 5 6 7 8 9 10

MOOD

☆☆☆☆☆

TODAY'S DIET

WATER INTAKE

BREAKFAST TIME : ....

CAL : .... CARBS: .... PROTEIN .... FAT ....

LUNCH TIME : ....

CAL : .... CARBS: .... PROTEIN .... FAT ....

DINNER TIME : ....

CAL : .... CARBS: .... PROTEIN .... FAT ....

SNACKS TIME: ....

CAL : .... CARBS: .... PROTEIN .... FAT ....

REACTION TO FOODS

MEAL : ....

FOOD : ....

SYMPTOMS

HOW MY APPETITE AFFECTED ?

1 2 3 4 5 6 7 8 9 10

NOT AFFECTED NO APPETITE

HOW IS MY URINATION

1 2 3 4 5 6 7 8 9 10

GOOD WORST

HOW IS MY BOWELS

1 2 3 4 5 6 7 8 9 10

CONSTIPATED LOOSE

EXACERBATING CONDITIONS

CURENT WEATHER

SUNNY OVERCAST

FOGGY

RAINY SNOWY

CURRENT WEATHER AFFECTING ME

1 2 3 4 5 6 7 8 9 10

NONE GREATLY

JOB STRESS LEVEL

1 2 3 4 5 6 7 8 9 10

LOW HIGH

TEMPERATURE

LOW HIGH

FAMILY HOME LIFE STRESS LEVEL

1 2 3 4 5 6 7 8 9 10

LOW HIGH

TOP 3 THINGS I WILL DO TO MY CARE-SELF TODAY

TOP 3 THINGS TO ACCOMPLISH TODAY

TOP 3 HIGHLIGHTS OF MY DAY

NOTES /COMMENTS

DATE: .... DAY: ....

DAILY QUOTE

"..
...."

	AM	PM
WEIGHT		
TEMPERATURE		
BLOOD PRESSURE		

SUGAR LEVEL

BEFORE BREAKFAST :	AFTER BREAKFAST:
BEFORE LUNCH :	AFTER LUNCH :
BEFORE DINNER :	AFTER DINNER :

BEDTIME :

SLEEP LAST NIGHT

☐ /HOURS

☐ ☺ ☐ ☹ ☐

NAPS TODAY

☐ /TOTAL HOURS ☐ /HOW MANY

DRUGS/VITAMINS /HERBS/MEDICATIONS	REASON	DOSAGE	TIME			REACTION

SYMPTOM NOTES

RECURRING SYMPTOMS	
NEW SYMPTOMS	

PAIN SITE IDENTIFICATION

MARK PAINFUL AREAS OF THE BODY

OVERALL MORNING PAIN LEVEL

1 2 3 4 5 6 7 8 9 10

LOW HIGH

OVERALL AFTERNOON PAIN LEVEL

1 2 3 4 5 6 7 8 9 10

LOW HIGH

OVERALL EVENING PAIN LEVEL

1 2 3 4 5 6 7 8 9 10

LOW HIGH

SUSPECTED TRIGGERS

....
....

MEDICATIONS: ....

DID THE MEDICATION HELP? ....

PHYSICAL ACTIVITY

ACTIVITY/ EXERCISE	DURATION	SETS	REPS	CAL	NOTES

FATIGUE

1 2 3 4 5 6 7 8 9 10

DEPRESSION / ANXIETY

1 2 3 4 5 6 7 8 9 10

MOOD

☆☆☆☆☆

TODAY'S DIET

WATER INTAKE

BREAKFAST TIME : ....

CAL : .... CARBS: .... PROTEIN .... FAT ....

LUNCH TIME : ....

CAL : .... CARBS: .... PROTEIN .... FAT ....

DINNER TIME : ....

CAL : .... CARBS: .... PROTEIN .... FAT ....

SNACKS TIME: ....

CAL : .... CARBS: .... PROTEIN .... FAT ....

REACTION TO FOODS

MEAL : ....

FOOD : ....

SYMPTOMS

HOW MY APPETITE AFFECTED ?

1 2 3 4 5 6 7 8 9 10

NOT AFFECTED NO APPETITE

HOW IS MY URINATION

1 2 3 4 5 6 7 8 9 10

GOOD WORST

HOW IS MY BOWELS

1 2 3 4 5 6 7 8 9 10

CONSTIPATED LOOSE

EXACERBATING CONDITIONS

CURENT WEATHER

SUNNY OVERCAST

FOGGY

RAINY SNOWY

CURRENT WEATHER AFFECTING ME

1 2 3 4 5 6 7 8 9 10

NONE GREATLY

JOB STRESS LEVEL

1 2 3 4 5 6 7 8 9 10

LOW HIGH

TEMPERATURE

LOW HIGH

FAMILY HOME LIFE STRESS LEVEL

1 2 3 4 5 6 7 8 9 10

LOW HIGH

TOP 3 THINGS I WILL DO TO MY CARE-SELF TODAY

TOP 3 THINGS TO ACCOMPLISH TODAY

TOP 3 HIGHLIGHTS OF MY DAY

NOTES /COMMENTS

DATE: .... DAY: ....

DAILY QUOTE

" ....
....
"

	AM	PM
WEIGHT		
TEMPERATURE		
BLOOD PRESSURE		

SUGAR LEVEL

BEFORE BREAKFAST :	AFTER BREAKFAST:
BEFORE LUNCH :	AFTER LUNCH :
BEFORE DINNER :	AFTER DINNER :

BEDTIME :

SLEEP LAST NIGHT

☐ /HOURS

☐ ☺ ☐ ☹ ☐

NAPS TODAY

☐ /TOTAL HOURS ☐ /HOW MANY

DRUGS/VITAMINS /HERBS/MEDICATIONS	REASON	DOSAGE	TIME			REACTION

SYMPTOM NOTES

RECURRING SYMPTOMS	
NEW SYMPTOMS	

PAIN SITE IDENTIFICATION

MARK PAINFUL AREAS OF THE BODY

OVERALL MORNING PAIN LEVEL

1 2 3 4 5 6 7 8 9 10

LOW HIGH

OVERALL EVENING PAIN LEVEL

1 2 3 4 5 6 7 8 9 10

LOW HIGH

OVERALL AFTERNOON PAIN LEVEL

1 2 3 4 5 6 7 8 9 10

LOW HIGH

SUSPECTED TRIGGERS

....
....

MEDICATIONS: ....

DID THE MEDICATION HELP? ....

PHYSICAL ACTIVITY

ACTIVITY/ EXERCISE	DURATION	SETS	REPS	CAL	NOTES

FATIGUE

1 2 3 4 5 6 7 8 9 10

DEPRESSION / ANXIETY

1 2 3 4 5 6 7 8 9 10

MOOD

☆☆☆☆☆

TODAY'S DIET

WATER INTAKE

BREAKFAST TIME : ....

....

....

....

....

CAL : .... CARBS: .... PROTEIN .... FAT ....

LUNCH TIME : ....

....

....

....

....

CAL : .... CARBS: .... PROTEIN .... FAT ....

DINNER TIME : ....

....

....

....

....

CAL : .... CARBS: .... PROTEIN .... FAT ....

SNACKS TIME: ....

....

....

....

....

CAL : .... CARBS: .... PROTEIN .... FAT ....

REACTION TO FOODS

MEAL : ....

FOOD : ....

SYMPTOMS

....

....

....

....

....

HOW MY APPETITE AFFECTED ?

1 2 3 4 5 6 7 8 9 10

NOT AFFECTED NO APPETITE

HOW IS MY URINATION

1 2 3 4 5 6 7 8 9 10

GOOD WORST

HOW IS MY BOWELS

1 2 3 4 5 6 7 8 9 10

CONSTIPATED LOOSE

EXACERBATING CONDITIONS

CURENT WEATHER

SUNNY OVERCAST

FOGGY

RAINY SNOWY

CURRENT WEATHER AFFECTING ME

1 2 3 4 5 6 7 8 9 10

NONE GREATLY

JOB STRESS LEVEL

1 2 3 4 5 6 7 8 9 10

LOW HIGH

TEMPERATURE

LOW HIGH

FAMILY HOME LIFE STRESS LEVEL

1 2 3 4 5 6 7 8 9 10

LOW HIGH

TOP 3 THINGS I WILL DO TO MY CARE-SELF TODAY

....

....

....

TOP 3 THINGS TO ACCOMPLISH TODAY

....

....

....

TOP 3 HIGHLIGHTS OF MY DAY

....

....

....

NOTES /COMMENTS

....

....

....

....

DATE: .... DAY: ....

DAILY QUOTE

"..
...."

	AM	PM
WEIGHT		
TEMPERATURE		
BLOOD PRESSURE		

SUGAR LEVEL

BEFORE BREAKFAST :	AFTER BREAKFAST:
BEFORE LUNCH :	AFTER LUNCH :
BEFORE DINNER :	AFTER DINNER :

BEDTIME :

SLEEP LAST NIGHT

☐ /HOURS

☐ ☐ ☐

NAPS TODAY

☐ /TOTAL HOURS ☐ /HOW MANY

DRUGS/VITAMINS /HERBS/MEDICATIONS	REASON	DOSAGE	TIME			REACTION

SYMPTOM NOTES

RECURRING SYMPTOMS	
NEW SYMPTOMS	

PAIN SITE IDENTIFICATION

MARK PAINFUL AREAS OF THE BODY

OVERALL MORNING PAIN LEVEL

1 2 3 4 5 6 7 8 9 10

LOW HIGH

OVERALL AFTERNOON PAIN LEVEL

1 2 3 4 5 6 7 8 9 10

LOW HIGH

OVERALL EVENING PAIN LEVEL

1 2 3 4 5 6 7 8 9 10

LOW HIGH

SUSPECTED TRIGGERS

....
....

MEDICATIONS: ....

DID THE MEDICATION HELP? ....

PHYSICAL ACTIVITY

ACTIVITY/ EXERCISE	DURATION	SETS	REPS	CAL	NOTES

FATIGUE

1 2 3 4 5 6 7 8 9 10

DEPRESSION / ANXIETY

1 2 3 4 5 6 7 8 9 10

MOOD

☆☆☆☆☆

TODAY'S DIET

WATER INTAKE

BREAKFAST TIME : ....

CAL : .... CARBS: .... PROTEIN .... FAT ....

LUNCH TIME : ....

CAL : .... CARBS: .... PROTEIN .... FAT ....

DINNER TIME : ....

CAL : .... CARBS: .... PROTEIN .... FAT ....

SNACKS TIME: ....

CAL : .... CARBS: .... PROTEIN .... FAT ....

REACTION TO FOODS

MEAL : ....

FOOD : ....

SYMPTOMS

....

HOW MY APPETITE AFFECTED ?

1 2 3 4 5 6 7 8 9 10

NOT AFFECTED NO APPETITE

HOW IS MY URINATION

1 2 3 4 5 6 7 8 9 10

GOOD WORST

HOW IS MY BOWELS

1 2 3 4 5 6 7 8 9 10

CONSTIPATED LOOSE

EXACERBATING CONDITIONS

CURENT WEATHER

SUNNY OVERCAST FOGGY RAINY SNOWY

CURRENT WEATHER AFFECTING ME

1 2 3 4 5 6 7 8 9 10

NONE GREATLY

JOB STRESS LEVEL

1 2 3 4 5 6 7 8 9 10

LOW HIGH

TEMPERATURE

LOW HIGH

FAMILY HOME LIFE STRESS LEVEL

1 2 3 4 5 6 7 8 9 10

LOW HIGH

TOP 3 THINGS I WILL DO TO MY CARE-SELF TODAY

....

TOP 3 THINGS TO ACCOMPLISH TODAY

....

TOP 3 HIGHLIGHTS OF MY DAY

....

NOTES /COMMENTS

....

DATE: .... DAY: ....

DAILY QUOTE

" ....
.... "

	AM	PM
WEIGHT		
TEMPERATURE		
BLOOD PRESSURE		

SUGAR LEVEL

BEFORE BREAKFAST :	AFTER BREAKFAST:
BEFORE LUNCH :	AFTER LUNCH :
BEFORE DINNER :	AFTER DINNER :
BEDTIME :	

SLEEP LAST NIGHT

☐ /HOURS

☐ ☺ ☐ ☹ ☐

NAPS TODAY

☐ /TOTAL HOURS ☐ /HOW MANY

DRUGS/VITAMINS /HERBS/MEDICATIONS	REASON	DOSAGE	TIME			REACTION

SYMPTOM NOTES

RECURRING SYMPTOMS	
NEW SYMPTOMS	

PAIN SITE IDENTIFICATION

MARK PAINFUL AREAS OF THE BODY

OVERALL MORNING PAIN LEVEL

1 2 3 4 5 6 7 8 9 10

LOW HIGH

OVERALL AFTERNOON PAIN LEVEL

1 2 3 4 5 6 7 8 9 10

LOW HIGH

OVERALL EVENING PAIN LEVEL

1 2 3 4 5 6 7 8 9 10

LOW HIGH

SUSPECTED TRIGGERS

....
....

MEDICATIONS: ....

DID THE MEDICATION HELP? ....

PHYSICAL ACTIVITY

ACTIVITY/ EXERCISE	DURATION	SETS	REPS	CAL	NOTES

FATIGUE

1 2 3 4 5 6 7 8 9 10

DEPRESSION / ANXIETY

1 2 3 4 5 6 7 8 9 10

MOOD

☆ ☆ ☆ ☆ ☆

TODAY'S DIET

WATER INTAKE

BREAKFAST TIME :

CAL : CARBS: PROTEIN FAT

LUNCH TIME :

CAL : CARBS: PROTEIN FAT

DINNER TIME :

CAL : CARBS: PROTEIN FAT

SNACKS TIME:

CAL : CARBS: PROTEIN FAT

REACTION TO FOODS

MEAL :

FOOD :

SYMPTOMS

HOW MY APPETITE AFFECTED ?

1 2 3 4 5 6 7 8 9 10

NOT AFFECTED NO APPETITE

HOW IS MY URINATION

1 2 3 4 5 6 7 8 9 10

GOOD WORST

HOW IS MY BOWELS

1 2 3 4 5 6 7 8 9 10

CONSTIPATED LOOSE

EXACERBATING CONDITIONS

CURENT WEATHER

SUNNY OVERCAST

FOGGY

RAINY SNOWY

CURRENT WEATHER AFFECTING ME

1 2 3 4 5 6 7 8 9 10

NONE GREATLY

JOB STRESS LEVEL

1 2 3 4 5 6 7 8 9 10

LOW HIGH

TEMPERATURE

LOW HIGH

FAMILY HOME LIFE STRESS LEVEL

1 2 3 4 5 6 7 8 9 10

LOW HIGH

TOP 3 THINGS I WILL DO TO MY CARE-SELF TODAY

TOP 3 THINGS TO ACCOMPLISH TODAY

TOP 3 HIGHLIGHTS OF MY DAY

NOTES /COMMENTS

DATE:.................... DAY: ....

DAILY QUOTE

"..
...."

	AM	PM
WEIGHT		
TEMPERATURE		
BLOOD PRESSURE		

SUGAR LEVEL

BEFORE BREAKFAST :	AFTER BREAKFAST:
BEFORE LUNCH :	AFTER LUNCH :
BEFORE DINNER :	AFTER DINNER :
BEDTIME :	

SLEEP LAST NIGHT

/HOURS

NAPS TODAY

/TOTAL HOURS /HOW MANY

DRUGS/VITAMINS /HERBS/MEDICATIONS	REASON	DOSAGE	TIME			REACTION

SYMPTOM NOTES

RECURRING SYMPTOMS	
NEW SYMPTOMS	

PAIN SITE IDENTIFICATION

MARK PAINFUL AREAS OF THE BODY

OVERALL MORNING PAIN LEVEL

1 2 3 4 5 6 7 8 9 10

LOW HIGH

OVERALL AFTERNOON PAIN LEVEL

1 2 3 4 5 6 7 8 9 10

LOW HIGH

OVERALL EVENING PAIN LEVEL

1 2 3 4 5 6 7 8 9 10

LOW HIGH

SUSPECTED TRIGGERS

....
....

MEDICATIONS: ....

DID THE MEDICATION HELP? ....

PHYSICAL ACTIVITY

ACTIVITY/ EXERCISE	DURATION	SETS	REPS	CAL	NOTES

FATIGUE

1 2 3 4 5 6 7 8 9 10

DEPRESSION / ANXIETY

1 2 3 4 5 6 7 8 9 10

MOOD

☆☆☆☆☆

TODAY'S DIET

WATER INTAKE

BREAKFAST TIME : ....

CAL : .... CARBS: .... PROTEIN .... FAT ....

LUNCH TIME : ....

CAL : .... CARBS: .... PROTEIN .... FAT ....

DINNER TIME : ....

CAL : .... CARBS: .... PROTEIN .... FAT ....

SNACKS TIME: ....

CAL : .... CARBS: .... PROTEIN .... FAT ....

REACTION TO FOODS

MEAL : ....

FOOD : ....

SYMPTOMS

HOW MY APPETITE AFFECTED ?

1 2 3 4 5 6 7 8 9 10

NOT AFFECTED NO APPETITE

HOW IS MY URINATION

1 2 3 4 5 6 7 8 9 10

GOOD WORST

HOW IS MY BOWELS

1 2 3 4 5 6 7 8 9 10

CONSTIPATED LOOSE

EXACERBATING CONDITIONS

CURENT WEATHER

SUNNY OVERCAST

FOGGY

RAINY SNOWY

CURRENT WEATHER AFFECTING ME

1 2 3 4 5 6 7 8 9 10

NONE GREATLY

JOB STRESS LEVEL

1 2 3 4 5 6 7 8 9 10

LOW HIGH

TEMPERATURE

LOW HIGH

FAMILY HOME LIFE STRESS LEVEL

1 2 3 4 5 6 7 8 9 10

LOW HIGH

TOP 3 THINGS I WILL DO TO MY CARE-SELF TODAY

TOP 3 THINGS TO ACCOMPLISH TODAY

TOP 3 HIGHLIGHTS OF MY DAY

NOTES /COMMENTS

DATE: .... **DAY:** ....

DAILY QUOTE

"..
...."

	AM	PM
WEIGHT		
TEMPERATURE		
BLOOD PRESSURE		

SUGAR LEVEL

BEFORE BREAKFAST :	AFTER BREAKFAST:
BEFORE LUNCH :	AFTER LUNCH :
BEFORE DINNER :	AFTER DINNER :

BEDTIME :

SLEEP LAST NIGHT

☐ /HOURS

☐ ☺ ☐ ☹ ☐

NAPS TODAY

☐ /TOTAL HOURS ☐ /HOW MANY

DRUGS/VITAMINS /HERBS/MEDICATIONS	REASON	DOSAGE	TIME			REACTION

SYMPTOM NOTES

RECURRING SYMPTOMS	
NEW SYMPTOMS	

PAIN SITE IDENTIFICATION

MARK PAINFUL AREAS OF THE BODY

OVERALL MORNING PAIN LEVEL

1 2 3 4 5 6 7 8 9 10

LOW HIGH

OVERALL EVENING PAIN LEVEL

1 2 3 4 5 6 7 8 9 10

LOW HIGH

OVERALL AFTERNOON PAIN LEVEL

1 2 3 4 5 6 7 8 9 10

LOW HIGH

SUSPECTED TRIGGERS

....
....

MEDICATIONS: ....

DID THE MEDICATION HELP? ....

PHYSICAL ACTIVITY

ACTIVITY/ EXERCISE	DURATION	SETS	REPS	CAL	NOTES

FATIGUE

1 2 3 4 5 6 7 8 9 10

DEPRESSION / ANXIETY

1 2 3 4 5 6 7 8 9 10

MOOD

☆☆☆☆☆

TODAY'S DIET

WATER INTAKE

BREAKFAST TIME : ....

....

....

....

....

CAL : .... CARBS: .... PROTEIN .... FAT ....

LUNCH TIME : ....

....

....

....

....

CAL : .... CARBS: .... PROTEIN .... FAT ....

DINNER TIME : ....

....

....

....

....

CAL : .... CARBS: .... PROTEIN .... FAT ....

SNACKS TIME: ....

....

....

....

....

CAL : .... CARBS: .... PROTEIN .... FAT ....

REACTION TO FOODS

MEAL : ....

FOOD : ....

SYMPTOMS

....

....

....

....

....

HOW MY APPETITE AFFECTED ?

1 2 3 4 5 6 7 8 9 10

NOT AFFECTED NO APPETITE

HOW IS MY URINATION

1 2 3 4 5 6 7 8 9 10

GOOD WORST

HOW IS MY BOWELS

1 2 3 4 5 6 7 8 9 10

CONSTIPATED LOOSE

EXACERBATING CONDITIONS

CURENT WEATHER

SUNNY OVERCAST

FOGGY

RAINY SNOWY

CURRENT WEATHER AFFECTING ME

1 2 3 4 5 6 7 8 9 10

NONE GREATLY

JOB STRESS LEVEL

1 2 3 4 5 6 7 8 9 10

LOW HIGH

TEMPERATURE

LOW HIGH

FAMILY HOME LIFE STRESS LEVEL

1 2 3 4 5 6 7 8 9 10

LOW HIGH

TOP 3 THINGS I WILL DO TO MY CARE-SELF TODAY

....

....

....

TOP 3 THINGS TO ACCOMPLISH TODAY

....

....

....

TOP 3 HIGHLIGHTS OF MY DAY

....

....

....

NOTES /COMMENTS

....

....

....

....

DATE: .... DAY: ....

DAILY QUOTE

"..

...."

	AM	PM
WEIGHT		
TEMPERATURE		
BLOOD PRESSURE		

SUGAR LEVEL

BEFORE BREAKFAST :	AFTER BREAKFAST:
BEFORE LUNCH :	AFTER LUNCH :
BEFORE DINNER :	AFTER DINNER :
BEDTIME :	

SLEEP LAST NIGHT

☐ /HOURS

☐ ☺ ☐ ☹ ☐ 😫

NAPS TODAY

☐ /TOTAL HOURS ☐ /HOW MANY

DRUGS/VITAMINS /HERBS/MEDICATIONS	REASON	DOSAGE	TIME			REACTION

SYMPTOM NOTES

RECURRING SYMPTOMS	
NEW SYMPTOMS	

PAIN SITE IDENTIFICATION

MARK PAINFUL AREAS OF THE BODY

OVERALL MORNING PAIN LEVEL

1 2 3 4 5 6 7 8 9 10

LOW HIGH

OVERALL AFTERNOON PAIN LEVEL

1 2 3 4 5 6 7 8 9 10

LOW HIGH

OVERALL EVENING PAIN LEVEL

1 2 3 4 5 6 7 8 9 10

LOW HIGH

SUSPECTED TRIGGERS

....

....

MEDICATIONS: ....

DID THE MEDICATION HELP? ....

PHYSICAL ACTIVITY

ACTIVITY/ EXERCISE	DURATION	SETS	REPS	CAL	NOTES

FATIGUE

1 2 3 4 5 6 7 8 9 10

DEPRESSION / ANXIETY

1 2 3 4 5 6 7 8 9 10

MOOD

☆ ☆ ☆ ☆ ☆

TODAY'S DIET

WATER INTAKE

BREAKFAST TIME : ....

CAL : .... CARBS: .... PROTEIN .... FAT ....

LUNCH TIME : ....

CAL : .... CARBS: .... PROTEIN .... FAT ....

DINNER TIME : ....

CAL : .... CARBS: .... PROTEIN .... FAT ....

SNACKS TIME: ....

CAL : .... CARBS: .... PROTEIN .... FAT ....

REACTION TO FOODS

MEAL : ....

FOOD : ....

SYMPTOMS

....

HOW MY APPETITE AFFECTED ?

1 2 3 4 5 6 7 8 9 10

NOT AFFECTED NO APPETITE

HOW IS MY URINATION

1 2 3 4 5 6 7 8 9 10

GOOD WORST

HOW IS MY BOWELS

1 2 3 4 5 6 7 8 9 10

CONSTIPATED LOOSE

EXACERBATING CONDITIONS

CURENT WEATHER

SUNNY OVERCAST

FOGGY

RAINY SNOWY

CURRENT WEATHER AFFECTING ME

1 2 3 4 5 6 7 8 9 10

NONE GREATLY

JOB STRESS LEVEL

1 2 3 4 5 6 7 8 9 10

LOW HIGH

TEMPERATURE

LOW HIGH

FAMILY HOME LIFE STRESS LEVEL

1 2 3 4 5 6 7 8 9 10

LOW HIGH

TOP 3 THINGS I WILL DO TO MY CARE-SELF TODAY

....

TOP 3 THINGS TO ACCOMPLISH TODAY

....

TOP 3 HIGHLIGHTS OF MY DAY

....

NOTES /COMMENTS

....

DATE: .... DAY: ....

DAILY QUOTE

"..
...."

	AM	PM
WEIGHT		
TEMPERATURE		
BLOOD PRESSURE		

SUGAR LEVEL

BEFORE BREAKFAST :	AFTER BREAKFAST:
BEFORE LUNCH :	AFTER LUNCH :
BEFORE DINNER :	AFTER DINNER :
BEDTIME :	

SLEEP LAST NIGHT

☐ /HOURS

☐ ☺ ☐ ☹ ☐

NAPS TODAY

☐ /TOTAL HOURS ☐ /HOW MANY

DRUGS/VITAMINS /HERBS/MEDICATIONS	REASON	DOSAGE	TIME			REACTION

SYMPTOM NOTES

RECURRING SYMPTOMS	
NEW SYMPTOMS	

PAIN SITE IDENTIFICATION

MARK PAINFUL AREAS OF THE BODY

OVERALL MORNING PAIN LEVEL

1 2 3 4 5 6 7 8 9 10

LOW HIGH

OVERALL AFTERNOON PAIN LEVEL

1 2 3 4 5 6 7 8 9 10

LOW HIGH

OVERALL EVENING PAIN LEVEL

1 2 3 4 5 6 7 8 9 10

LOW HIGH

SUSPECTED TRIGGERS

....
....

MEDICATIONS: ....

DID THE MEDICATION HELP? ....

PHYSICAL ACTIVITY

ACTIVITY/ EXERCISE	DURATION	SETS	REPS	CAL	NOTES

FATIGUE

1 2 3 4 5 6 7 8 9 10

DEPRESSION / ANXIETY

1 2 3 4 5 6 7 8 9 10

MOOD

☆ ☆ ☆ ☆ ☆

TODAY'S DIET

WATER INTAKE

BREAKFAST

TIME : ....

CAL : .... CARBS: .... PROTEIN .... FAT ....

LUNCH

TIME : ....

CAL : .... CARBS: .... PROTEIN .... FAT ....

DINNER

TIME : ....

CAL : .... CARBS: .... PROTEIN .... FAT ....

SNACKS

TIME: ....

CAL : .... CARBS: .... PROTEIN .... FAT ....

REACTION TO FOODS

MEAL : ....

FOOD : ....

SYMPTOMS

HOW MY APPETITE AFFECTED ?

1 2 3 4 5 6 7 8 9 10

NOT AFFECTED NO APPETITE

HOW IS MY URINATION

1 2 3 4 5 6 7 8 9 10

GOOD WORST

HOW IS MY BOWELS

1 2 3 4 5 6 7 8 9 10

CONSTIPATED LOOSE

EXACERBATING CONDITIONS

CURENT WEATHER

SUNNY OVERCAST FOGGY RAINY SNOWY

CURRENT WEATHER AFFECTING ME

1 2 3 4 5 6 7 8 9 10

NONE GREATLY

JOB STRESS LEVEL

1 2 3 4 5 6 7 8 9 10

LOW HIGH

TEMPERATURE

LOW HIGH

FAMILY HOME LIFE STRESS LEVEL

1 2 3 4 5 6 7 8 9 10

LOW HIGH

TOP 3 THINGS I WILL DO TO MY CARE-SELF TODAY

TOP 3 THINGS TO ACCOMPLISH TODAY

TOP 3 HIGHLIGHTS OF MY DAY

NOTES /COMMENTS

DATE: .... DAY: ....

DAILY QUOTE

"..

...."

	AM	PM
WEIGHT		
TEMPERATURE		
BLOOD PRESSURE		

SUGAR LEVEL

BEFORE BREAKFAST :	AFTER BREAKFAST:
BEFORE LUNCH :	AFTER LUNCH :
BEFORE DINNER :	AFTER DINNER :
BEDTIME :	

SLEEP LAST NIGHT

☐ /HOURS

☐ ☺ ☐ ☹ ☐ 😫

NAPS TODAY

☐ /TOTAL HOURS ☐ /HOW MANY

DRUGS/VITAMINS /HERBS/MEDICATIONS	REASON	DOSAGE	TIME			REACTION

SYMPTOM NOTES

RECURRING SYMPTOMS	
NEW SYMPTOMS	

PAIN SITE IDENTIFICATION

MARK PAINFUL AREAS OF THE BODY

OVERALL MORNING PAIN LEVEL

1 2 3 4 5 6 7 8 9 10

LOW HIGH

OVERALL AFTERNOON PAIN LEVEL

1 2 3 4 5 6 7 8 9 10

LOW HIGH

OVERALL EVENING PAIN LEVEL

1 2 3 4 5 6 7 8 9 10

LOW HIGH

SUSPECTED TRIGGERS

....

....

MEDICATIONS: ....

DID THE MEDICATION HELP? ....

PHYSICAL ACTIVITY

ACTIVITY/ EXERCISE	DURATION	SETS	REPS	CAL	NOTES

FATIGUE

1 2 3 4 5 6 7 8 9 10

DEPRESSION / ANXIETY

1 2 3 4 5 6 7 8 9 10

MOOD

☆☆☆☆☆

TODAY'S DIET

WATER INTAKE

BREAKFAST TIME : ....

....

....

....

CAL : .... CARBS: .... PROTEIN .... FAT ....

LUNCH TIME : ....

....

....

....

CAL : .... CARBS: .... PROTEIN .... FAT ....

DINNER TIME : ....

....

....

....

CAL : .... CARBS: .... PROTEIN .... FAT ....

SNACKS TIME: ....

....

....

....

CAL : .... CARBS: .... PROTEIN .... FAT ....

REACTION TO FOODS

MEAL : ....

FOOD : ....

SYMPTOMS

....

....

....

....

....

HOW MY APPETITE AFFECTED ?

1 2 3 4 5 6 7 8 9 10

NOT AFFECTED NO APPETITE

HOW IS MY URINATION

1 2 3 4 5 6 7 8 9 10

GOOD WORST

HOW IS MY BOWELS

1 2 3 4 5 6 7 8 9 10

CONSTIPATED LOOSE

EXACERBATING CONDITIONS

CURENT WEATHER

SUNNY OVERCAST

FOGGY

RAINY SNOWY

CURRENT WEATHER AFFECTING ME

1 2 3 4 5 6 7 8 9 10

NONE GREATLY

JOB STRESS LEVEL

1 2 3 4 5 6 7 8 9 10

LOW HIGH

TEMPERATURE

LOW HIGH

FAMILY HOME LIFE STRESS LEVEL

1 2 3 4 5 6 7 8 9 10

LOW HIGH

TOP 3 THINGS I WILL DO TO MY CARE-SELF TODAY

....

....

....

TOP 3 THINGS TO ACCOMPLISH TODAY

....

....

....

TOP 3 HIGHLIGHTS OF MY DAY

....

....

....

NOTES /COMMENTS

....

....

....

....

DATE:.................... DAY: ....

DAILY QUOTE

"..
...."

	AM	PM
WEIGHT		
TEMPERATURE		
BLOOD PRESSURE		

SUGAR LEVEL

BEFORE BREAKFAST :	AFTER BREAKFAST:
BEFORE LUNCH :	AFTER LUNCH :
BEFORE DINNER :	AFTER DINNER :

BEDTIME :

SLEEP LAST NIGHT

☐ /HOURS

☐ ☺ ☐ ☹ ☐ 😫

NAPS TODAY

☐ /TOTAL HOURS ☐ /HOW MANY

DRUGS/VITAMINS /HERBS/MEDICATIONS	REASON	DOSAGE	TIME			REACTION

SYMPTOM NOTES

RECURRING SYMPTOMS	
NEW SYMPTOMS	

PAIN SITE IDENTIFICATION

MARK PAINFUL AREAS OF THE BODY

OVERALL MORNING PAIN LEVEL

1 2 3 4 5 6 7 8 9 10

LOW HIGH

OVERALL EVENING PAIN LEVEL

1 2 3 4 5 6 7 8 9 10

LOW HIGH

OVERALL AFTERNOON PAIN LEVEL

1 2 3 4 5 6 7 8 9 10

LOW HIGH

SUSPECTED TRIGGERS

....
....

MEDICATIONS: ....

DID THE MEDICATION HELP? ....

PHYSICAL ACTIVITY

ACTIVITY/ EXERCISE	DURATION	SETS	REPS	CAL	NOTES

FATIGUE

1 2 3 4 5 6 7 8 9 10

DEPRESSION / ANXIETY

1 2 3 4 5 6 7 8 9 10

MOOD

☆☆☆☆☆

TODAY'S DIET

WATER INTAKE

BREAKFAST TIME : ....

CAL : .... CARBS: .... PROTEIN .... FAT ....

LUNCH TIME : ....

CAL : .... CARBS: .... PROTEIN .... FAT ....

DINNER TIME : ....

CAL : .... CARBS: .... PROTEIN .... FAT ....

SNACKS TIME: ....

CAL : .... CARBS: .... PROTEIN .... FAT ....

REACTION TO FOODS

MEAL : ....

FOOD : ....

SYMPTOMS

HOW MY APPETITE AFFECTED ?

1 2 3 4 5 6 7 8 9 10

NOT AFFECTED NO APPETITE

HOW IS MY URINATION

1 2 3 4 5 6 7 8 9 10

GOOD WORST

HOW IS MY BOWELS

1 2 3 4 5 6 7 8 9 10

CONSTIPATED LOOSE

EXACERBATING CONDITIONS

CURENT WEATHER

SUNNY OVERCAST

FOGGY

RAINY SNOWY

CURRENT WEATHER AFFECTING ME

1 2 3 4 5 6 7 8 9 10

NONE GREATLY

JOB STRESS LEVEL

1 2 3 4 5 6 7 8 9 10

LOW HIGH

TEMPERATURE

LOW HIGH

FAMILY HOME LIFE STRESS LEVEL

1 2 3 4 5 6 7 8 9 10

LOW HIGH

TOP 3 THINGS I WILL DO TO MY CARE-SELF TODAY

TOP 3 THINGS TO ACCOMPLISH TODAY

TOP 3 HIGHLIGHTS OF MY DAY

NOTES /COMMENTS

DATE: .... DAY: ....

DAILY QUOTE

" ....
....
"

	AM	PM
WEIGHT		
TEMPERATURE		
BLOOD PRESSURE		

SUGAR LEVEL

BEFORE BREAKFAST :	AFTER BREAKFAST:
BEFORE LUNCH :	AFTER LUNCH :
BEFORE DINNER :	AFTER DINNER :

BEDTIME :

SLEEP LAST NIGHT

☐ /HOURS

☐ ☺ ☐ ☹ ☐

NAPS TODAY

☐ /TOTAL HOURS ☐ /HOW MANY

DRUGS/VITAMINS /HERBS/MEDICATIONS	REASON	DOSAGE	TIME			REACTION

SYMPTOM NOTES

RECURRING SYMPTOMS	
NEW SYMPTOMS	

PAIN SITE IDENTIFICATION

MARK PAINFUL AREAS OF THE BODY

OVERALL MORNING PAIN LEVEL

1 2 3 4 5 6 7 8 9 10

LOW HIGH

OVERALL AFTERNOON PAIN LEVEL

1 2 3 4 5 6 7 8 9 10

LOW HIGH

OVERALL EVENING PAIN LEVEL

1 2 3 4 5 6 7 8 9 10

LOW HIGH

SUSPECTED TRIGGERS

....
....

MEDICATIONS: ....

DID THE MEDICATION HELP? ....

PHYSICAL ACTIVITY

ACTIVITY/ EXERCISE	DURATION	SETS	REPS	CAL	NOTES

FATIGUE

1 2 3 4 5 6 7 8 9 10

DEPRESSION / ANXIETY

1 2 3 4 5 6 7 8 9 10

MOOD

☆☆☆☆☆

TODAY'S DIET

WATER INTAKE

BREAKFAST TIME : ....

....
....
....

CAL : .... CARBS: .... PROTEIN .... FAT ....

LUNCH TIME : ....

....
....
....

CAL : .... CARBS: .... PROTEIN .... FAT ....

DINNER TIME : ....

....
....
....

CAL : .... CARBS: .... PROTEIN .... FAT ....

SNACKS TIME: ....

....
....
....

CAL : .... CARBS: .... PROTEIN .... FAT ....

REACTION TO FOODS

MEAL : ....

FOOD : ....

SYMPTOMS

....
....
....
....
....

HOW MY APPETITE AFFECTED ?

1 2 3 4 5 6 7 8 9 10

NOT AFFECTED NO APPETITE

HOW IS MY URINATION

1 2 3 4 5 6 7 8 9 10

GOOD WORST

HOW IS MY BOWELS

1 2 3 4 5 6 7 8 9 10

CONSTIPATED LOOSE

EXACERBATING CONDITIONS

CURENT WEATHER

SUNNY OVERCAST

FOGGY

RAINY SNOWY

CURRENT WEATHER AFFECTING ME

1 2 3 4 5 6 7 8 9 10

NONE GREATLY

JOB STRESS LEVEL

1 2 3 4 5 6 7 8 9 10

LOW HIGH

TEMPERATURE

LOW HIGH

FAMILY HOME LIFE STRESS LEVEL

1 2 3 4 5 6 7 8 9 10

LOW HIGH

TOP 3 THINGS I WILL DO TO MY CARE-SELF TODAY

....
....
....

TOP 3 THINGS TO ACCOMPLISH TODAY

....
....
....

TOP 3 HIGHLIGHTS OF MY DAY

....
....
....

NOTES /COMMENTS

....
....
....
....

DATE: .... DAY: ....

DAILY QUOTE

" ....
.... "

	AM	PM
WEIGHT		
TEMPERATURE		
BLOOD PRESSURE		

SUGAR LEVEL

BEFORE BREAKFAST :	AFTER BREAKFAST:
BEFORE LUNCH :	AFTER LUNCH :
BEFORE DINNER :	AFTER DINNER :
BEDTIME :	

SLEEP LAST NIGHT

☐ /HOURS

☐ ☺ ☐ ☹ ☐ 😫

NAPS TODAY

☐ /TOTAL HOURS ☐ /HOW MANY

DRUGS/VITAMINS /HERBS/MEDICATIONS	REASON	DOSAGE	TIME			REACTION

SYMPTOM NOTES

RECURRING SYMPTOMS	
NEW SYMPTOMS	

PAIN SITE IDENTIFICATION

MARK PAINFUL AREAS OF THE BODY

OVERALL MORNING PAIN LEVEL

1 2 3 4 5 6 7 8 9 10

LOW HIGH

OVERALL AFTERNOON PAIN LEVEL

1 2 3 4 5 6 7 8 9 10

LOW HIGH

OVERALL EVENING PAIN LEVEL

1 2 3 4 5 6 7 8 9 10

LOW HIGH

SUSPECTED TRIGGERS

....
....

MEDICATIONS: ....

DID THE MEDICATION HELP? ....

PHYSICAL ACTIVITY

ACTIVITY/ EXERCISE	DURATION	SETS	REPS	CAL	NOTES

FATIGUE

1 2 3 4 5 6 7 8 9 10

DEPRESSION / ANXIETY

1 2 3 4 5 6 7 8 9 10

MOOD

☆ ☆ ☆ ☆ ☆

TODAY'S DIET

WATER INTAKE

BREAKFAST
TIME : ....

CAL : .... CARBS: .... PROTEIN .... FAT ....

LUNCH
TIME : ....

CAL : .... CARBS: .... PROTEIN .... FAT ....

DINNER
TIME : ....

CAL : .... CARBS: .... PROTEIN .... FAT ....

SNACKS
TIME: ....

CAL : .... CARBS: .... PROTEIN .... FAT ....

REACTION TO FOODS

MEAL : ....

FOOD : ....

SYMPTOMS

HOW MY APPETITE AFFECTED ?
1 2 3 4 5 6 7 8 9 10

NOT AFFECTED NO APPETITE

HOW IS MY URINATION
1 2 3 4 5 6 7 8 9 10

GOOD WORST

HOW IS MY BOWELS
1 2 3 4 5 6 7 8 9 10

CONSTIPATED LOOSE

EXACERBATING CONDITIONS

CURENT WEATHER

SUNNY OVERCAST

FOGGY

RAINY SNOWY

CURRENT WEATHER AFFECTING ME

1 2 3 4 5 6 7 8 9 10

NONE GREATLY

JOB STRESS LEVEL

1 2 3 4 5 6 7 8 9 10

LOW HIGH

TEMPERATURE

LOW HIGH

FAMILY HOME LIFE STRESS LEVEL

1 2 3 4 5 6 7 8 9 10

LOW HIGH

TOP 3 THINGS I WILL DO TO MY CARE-SELF TODAY

TOP 3 THINGS TO ACCOMPLISH TODAY

TOP 3 HIGHLIGHTS OF MY DAY

NOTES /COMMENTS

DATE: .... DAY: ....

DAILY QUOTE

"..
...."

	AM	PM
WEIGHT		
TEMPERATURE		
BLOOD PRESSURE		

SUGAR LEVEL

BEFORE BREAKFAST :	AFTER BREAKFAST:
BEFORE LUNCH :	AFTER LUNCH :
BEFORE DINNER :	AFTER DINNER :
BEDTIME :	

SLEEP LAST NIGHT

☐ /HOURS

☐ ☺ ☐ ☹ ☐ 😫

NAPS TODAY

☐ /TOTAL HOURS ☐ /HOW MANY

DRUGS/VITAMINS /HERBS/MEDICATIONS	REASON	DOSAGE	TIME			REACTION

SYMPTOM NOTES

RECURRING SYMPTOMS	
NEW SYMPTOMS	

PAIN SITE IDENTIFICATION

MARK PAINFUL AREAS OF THE BODY

OVERALL MORNING PAIN LEVEL

1 2 3 4 5 6 7 8 9 10

LOW HIGH

OVERALL AFTERNOON PAIN LEVEL

1 2 3 4 5 6 7 8 9 10

LOW HIGH

OVERALL EVENING PAIN LEVEL

1 2 3 4 5 6 7 8 9 10

LOW HIGH

SUSPECTED TRIGGERS

....
....

MEDICATIONS: ....

DID THE MEDICATION HELP? ....

PHYSICAL ACTIVITY

ACTIVITY/ EXERCISE	DURATION	SETS	REPS	CAL	NOTES

FATIGUE

1 2 3 4 5 6 7 8 9 10

DEPRESSION / ANXIETY

1 2 3 4 5 6 7 8 9 10

MOOD

☆ ☆ ☆ ☆ ☆

TODAY'S DIET

WATER INTAKE

BREAKFAST TIME :

CAL : CARBS: PROTEIN FAT

LUNCH TIME :

CAL : CARBS: PROTEIN FAT

DINNER TIME :

CAL : CARBS: PROTEIN FAT

SNACKS TIME:

CAL : CARBS: PROTEIN FAT

REACTION TO FOODS

MEAL :

FOOD :

SYMPTOMS

HOW MY APPETITE AFFECTED ?

1 2 3 4 5 6 7 8 9 10

NOT AFFECTED NO APPETITE

HOW IS MY URINATION

1 2 3 4 5 6 7 8 9 10

GOOD WORST

HOW IS MY BOWELS

1 2 3 4 5 6 7 8 9 10

CONSTIPATED LOOSE

EXACERBATING CONDITIONS

CURENT WEATHER

SUNNY OVERCAST

FOGGY

RAINY SNOWY

CURRENT WEATHER AFFECTING ME

1 2 3 4 5 6 7 8 9 10

NONE GREATLY

JOB STRESS LEVEL

1 2 3 4 5 6 7 8 9 10

LOW HIGH

TEMPERATURE

LOW HIGH

FAMILY HOME LIFE STRESS LEVEL

1 2 3 4 5 6 7 8 9 10

LOW HIGH

TOP 3 THINGS I WILL DO TO MY CARE-SELF TODAY

TOP 3 THINGS TO ACCOMPLISH TODAY

TOP 3 HIGHLIGHTS OF MY DAY

NOTES /COMMENTS

DATE: .... DAY: ....

DAILY QUOTE

" ....
.... "

	AM	PM
WEIGHT		
TEMPERATURE		
BLOOD PRESSURE		

SUGAR LEVEL

BEFORE BREAKFAST :	AFTER BREAKFAST:
BEFORE LUNCH :	AFTER LUNCH :
BEFORE DINNER :	AFTER DINNER :

BEDTIME :

SLEEP LAST NIGHT

☐ /HOURS

☐ ☺ ☐ ☹ ☐

NAPS TODAY

☐ /TOTAL HOURS ☐ /HOW MANY

DRUGS/VITAMINS /HERBS/MEDICATIONS	REASON	DOSAGE	TIME			REACTION

SYMPTOM NOTES

RECURRING SYMPTOMS	
NEW SYMPTOMS	

PAIN SITE IDENTIFICATION

MARK PAINFUL AREAS OF THE BODY

OVERALL MORNING PAIN LEVEL

1 2 3 4 5 6 7 8 9 10

LOW HIGH

OVERALL AFTERNOON PAIN LEVEL

1 2 3 4 5 6 7 8 9 10

LOW HIGH

OVERALL EVENING PAIN LEVEL

1 2 3 4 5 6 7 8 9 10

LOW HIGH

SUSPECTED TRIGGERS

....
....

MEDICATIONS: ....

DID THE MEDICATION HELP? ....

PHYSICAL ACTIVITY

ACTIVITY/ EXERCISE	DURATION	SETS	REPS	CAL	NOTES

FATIGUE

1 2 3 4 5 6 7 8 9 10

DEPRESSION / ANXIETY

1 2 3 4 5 6 7 8 9 10

MOOD

☆ ☆ ☆ ☆ ☆

TODAY'S DIET

WATER INTAKE

BREAKFAST TIME : ....

....

CAL : .... CARBS: .... PROTEIN .... FAT ....

LUNCH TIME : ....

....

CAL : .... CARBS: .... PROTEIN .... FAT ....

DINNER TIME : ....

....

CAL : .... CARBS: .... PROTEIN .... FAT ....

SNACKS TIME: ....

....

CAL : .... CARBS: .... PROTEIN .... FAT ....

REACTION TO FOODS

MEAL : ....

FOOD : ....

SYMPTOMS

....

HOW MY APPETITE AFFECTED ?

1 2 3 4 5 6 7 8 9 10

NOT AFFECTED NO APPETITE

HOW IS MY URINATION

1 2 3 4 5 6 7 8 9 10

GOOD WORST

HOW IS MY BOWELS

1 2 3 4 5 6 7 8 9 10

CONSTIPATED LOOSE

EXACERBATING CONDITIONS

CURENT WEATHER

SUNNY OVERCAST

FOGGY

RAINY SNOWY

CURRENT WEATHER AFFECTING ME

1 2 3 4 5 6 7 8 9 10

NONE GREATLY

JOB STRESS LEVEL

1 2 3 4 5 6 7 8 9 10

LOW HIGH

TEMPERATURE

LOW HIGH

FAMILY HOME LIFE STRESS LEVEL

1 2 3 4 5 6 7 8 9 10

LOW HIGH

TOP 3 THINGS I WILL DO TO MY CARE-SELF TODAY

....

TOP 3 THINGS TO ACCOMPLISH TODAY

....

TOP 3 HIGHLIGHTS OF MY DAY

....

NOTES /COMMENTS

....

DATE: .... DAY: ....

DAILY QUOTE

"..
...."

	AM	PM
WEIGHT		
TEMPERATURE		
BLOOD PRESSURE		

SUGAR LEVEL

BEFORE BREAKFAST :	AFTER BREAKFAST:
BEFORE LUNCH :	AFTER LUNCH :
BEFORE DINNER :	AFTER DINNER :
BEDTIME :	

SLEEP LAST NIGHT

☐ /HOURS

☐ ☺ ☐ ☹ ☐ 😫

NAPS TODAY

☐ /TOTAL HOURS ☐ /HOW MANY

DRUGS/VITAMINS /HERBS/MEDICATIONS	REASON	DOSAGE	TIME			REACTION

SYMPTOM NOTES	
RECURRING SYMPTOMS	
NEW SYMPTOMS	

PAIN SITE IDENTIFICATION

MARK PAINFUL AREAS OF THE BODY

OVERALL MORNING PAIN LEVEL

1 2 3 4 5 6 7 8 9 10

LOW HIGH

OVERALL AFTERNOON PAIN LEVEL

1 2 3 4 5 6 7 8 9 10

LOW HIGH

OVERALL EVENING PAIN LEVEL

1 2 3 4 5 6 7 8 9 10

LOW HIGH

SUSPECTED TRIGGERS

....
....

MEDICATIONS: ....

DID THE MEDICATION HELP? ....

PHYSICAL ACTIVITY

ACTIVITY/ EXERCISE	DURATION	SETS	REPS	CAL	NOTES

FATIGUE

1 2 3 4 5 6 7 8 9 10

DEPRESSION / ANXIETY

1 2 3 4 5 6 7 8 9 10

MOOD

☆ ☆ ☆ ☆ ☆

TODAY'S DIET

WATER INTAKE

BREAKFAST TIME : ....

....

CAL : .... CARBS: .... PROTEIN .... FAT ....

LUNCH TIME : ....

....

CAL : .... CARBS: .... PROTEIN .... FAT ....

DINNER TIME : ....

....

CAL : .... CARBS: .... PROTEIN .... FAT ....

SNACKS TIME: ....

....

CAL : .... CARBS: .... PROTEIN .... FAT ....

REACTION TO FOODS

MEAL : ....

FOOD : ....

SYMPTOMS

....

HOW MY APPETITE AFFECTED ?

1 2 3 4 5 6 7 8 9 10

NOT AFFECTED NO APPETITE

HOW IS MY URINATION

1 2 3 4 5 6 7 8 9 10

GOOD WORST

HOW IS MY BOWELS

1 2 3 4 5 6 7 8 9 10

CONSTIPATED LOOSE

EXACERBATING CONDITIONS

CURENT WEATHER

SUNNY OVERCAST FOGGY RAINY SNOWY

CURRENT WEATHER AFFECTING ME

1 2 3 4 5 6 7 8 9 10

NONE GREATLY

TEMPERATURE

LOW HIGH

JOB STRESS LEVEL

1 2 3 4 5 6 7 8 9 10

LOW HIGH

FAMILY HOME LIFE STRESS LEVEL

1 2 3 4 5 6 7 8 9 10

LOW HIGH

TOP 3 THINGS I WILL DO TO MY CARE-SELF TODAY

....

TOP 3 THINGS TO ACCOMPLISH TODAY

....

TOP 3 HIGHLIGHTS OF MY DAY

....

NOTES /COMMENTS

....

DATE: .... DAY: ....

DAILY QUOTE

"..
...."

	AM	PM
WEIGHT		
TEMPERATURE		
BLOOD PRESSURE		

SUGAR LEVEL

BEFORE BREAKFAST :	AFTER BREAKFAST:
BEFORE LUNCH :	AFTER LUNCH :
BEFORE DINNER :	AFTER DINNER :
BEDTIME :	

SLEEP LAST NIGHT

☐ /HOURS

☐ ☺ ☐ ☹ ☐ 😫

NAPS TODAY

☐ /TOTAL HOURS ☐ /HOW MANY

DRUGS/VITAMINS /HERBS/MEDICATIONS	REASON	DOSAGE	TIME			REACTION

SYMPTOM NOTES

RECURRING SYMPTOMS	
NEW SYMPTOMS	

PAIN SITE IDENTIFICATION

MARK PAINFUL AREAS OF THE BODY

OVERALL MORNING PAIN LEVEL

1 2 3 4 5 6 7 8 9 10

LOW HIGH

OVERALL AFTERNOON PAIN LEVEL

1 2 3 4 5 6 7 8 9 10

LOW HIGH

OVERALL EVENING PAIN LEVEL

1 2 3 4 5 6 7 8 9 10

LOW HIGH

SUSPECTED TRIGGERS

....
....

MEDICATIONS: ....

DID THE MEDICATION HELP? ....

PHYSICAL ACTIVITY

ACTIVITY/ EXERCISE	DURATION	SETS	REPS	CAL	NOTES

FATIGUE

1 2 3 4 5 6 7 8 9 10

DEPRESSION / ANXIETY

1 2 3 4 5 6 7 8 9 10

MOOD

☆☆☆☆☆

TODAY'S DIET

WATER INTAKE

BREAKFAST TIME : ....

CAL : .... CARBS: .... PROTEIN .... FAT ....

LUNCH TIME : ....

CAL : .... CARBS: .... PROTEIN .... FAT ....

DINNER TIME : ....

CAL : .... CARBS: .... PROTEIN .... FAT ....

SNACKS TIME: ....

CAL : .... CARBS: .... PROTEIN .... FAT ....

REACTION TO FOODS

MEAL : ....

FOOD : ....

SYMPTOMS

....

HOW MY APPETITE AFFECTED ?

1 2 3 4 5 6 7 8 9 10

NOT AFFECTED NO APPETITE

HOW IS MY URINATION

1 2 3 4 5 6 7 8 9 10

GOOD WORST

HOW IS MY BOWELS

1 2 3 4 5 6 7 8 9 10

CONSTIPATED LOOSE

EXACERBATING CONDITIONS

CURENT WEATHER

SUNNY OVERCAST FOGGY RAINY SNOWY

CURRENT WEATHER AFFECTING ME

1 2 3 4 5 6 7 8 9 10

NONE GREATLY

JOB STRESS LEVEL

1 2 3 4 5 6 7 8 9 10

LOW HIGH

TEMPERATURE

LOW HIGH

FAMILY HOME LIFE STRESS LEVEL

1 2 3 4 5 6 7 8 9 10

LOW HIGH

TOP 3 THINGS I WILL DO TO MY CARE-SELF TODAY

....

TOP 3 THINGS TO ACCOMPLISH TODAY

....

TOP 3 HIGHLIGHTS OF MY DAY

....

NOTES /COMMENTS

....

DATE: .... DAY: ....

DAILY QUOTE

"..
...."

	AM	PM
WEIGHT		
TEMPERATURE		
BLOOD PRESSURE		

SUGAR LEVEL

BEFORE BREAKFAST :	AFTER BREAKFAST:
BEFORE LUNCH :	AFTER LUNCH :
BEFORE DINNER :	AFTER DINNER :
BEDTIME :	

SLEEP LAST NIGHT

☐ /HOURS

☐ ☺ ☐ ☹ ☐

NAPS TODAY

☐ /TOTAL HOURS ☐ /HOW MANY

DRUGS/VITAMINS /HERBS/MEDICATIONS	REASON	DOSAGE	TIME			REACTION

SYMPTOM NOTES

RECURRING SYMPTOMS	
NEW SYMPTOMS	

PAIN SITE IDENTIFICATION

MARK PAINFUL AREAS OF THE BODY

OVERALL MORNING PAIN LEVEL

1 2 3 4 5 6 7 8 9 10

LOW HIGH

OVERALL AFTERNOON PAIN LEVEL

1 2 3 4 5 6 7 8 9 10

LOW HIGH

OVERALL EVENING PAIN LEVEL

1 2 3 4 5 6 7 8 9 10

LOW HIGH

SUSPECTED TRIGGERS

....
....

MEDICATIONS: ....

DID THE MEDICATION HELP? ....

PHYSICAL ACTIVITY

ACTIVITY/ EXERCISE	DURATION	SETS	REPS	CAL	NOTES

FATIGUE

1 2 3 4 5 6 7 8 9 10

DEPRESSION / ANXIETY

1 2 3 4 5 6 7 8 9 10

MOOD

☆ ☆ ☆ ☆ ☆

TODAY'S DIET

WATER INTAKE

BREAKFAST TIME : ....

CAL : .... CARBS: .... PROTEIN .... FAT ....

LUNCH TIME : ....

CAL : .... CARBS: .... PROTEIN .... FAT ....

DINNER TIME : ....

CAL : .... CARBS: .... PROTEIN .... FAT ....

SNACKS TIME: ....

CAL : .... CARBS: .... PROTEIN .... FAT ....

REACTION TO FOODS

MEAL : ....

FOOD : ....

SYMPTOMS

HOW MY APPETITE AFFECTED ?

1 2 3 4 5 6 7 8 9 10

NOT AFFECTED NO APPETITE

HOW IS MY URINATION

1 2 3 4 5 6 7 8 9 10

GOOD WORST

HOW IS MY BOWELS

1 2 3 4 5 6 7 8 9 10

CONSTIPATED LOOSE

EXACERBATING CONDITIONS

CURENT WEATHER

SUNNY OVERCAST

FOGGY

RAINY SNOWY

CURRENT WEATHER AFFECTING ME

1 2 3 4 5 6 7 8 9 10

NONE GREATLY

JOB STRESS LEVEL

1 2 3 4 5 6 7 8 9 10

LOW HIGH

TEMPERATURE

LOW HIGH

FAMILY HOME LIFE STRESS LEVEL

1 2 3 4 5 6 7 8 9 10

LOW HIGH

TOP 3 THINGS I WILL DO TO MY CARE-SELF TODAY

TOP 3 THINGS TO ACCOMPLISH TODAY

TOP 3 HIGHLIGHTS OF MY DAY

NOTES /COMMENTS

DATE: .... DAY: ....

DAILY QUOTE

"..
...."

	AM	PM
WEIGHT		
TEMPERATURE		
BLOOD PRESSURE		

SUGAR LEVEL

BEFORE BREAKFAST :	AFTER BREAKFAST:
BEFORE LUNCH :	AFTER LUNCH :
BEFORE DINNER :	AFTER DINNER :

BEDTIME :

SLEEP LAST NIGHT

☐ /HOURS

☐ ☺ ☐ ☹ ☐

NAPS TODAY

☐ /TOTAL HOURS ☐ /HOW MANY

DRUGS/VITAMINS /HERBS/MEDICATIONS	REASON	DOSAGE	TIME			REACTION

SYMPTOM NOTES

RECURRING SYMPTOMS	
NEW SYMPTOMS	

PAIN SITE IDENTIFICATION

MARK PAINFUL AREAS OF THE BODY

OVERALL MORNING PAIN LEVEL

1 2 3 4 5 6 7 8 9 10

LOW HIGH

OVERALL EVENING PAIN LEVEL

1 2 3 4 5 6 7 8 9 10

LOW HIGH

OVERALL AFTERNOON PAIN LEVEL

1 2 3 4 5 6 7 8 9 10

LOW HIGH

SUSPECTED TRIGGERS

....
....

MEDICATIONS: ....

DID THE MEDICATION HELP? ....

PHYSICAL ACTIVITY

ACTIVITY/ EXERCISE	DURATION	SETS	REPS	CAL	NOTES

FATIGUE

1 2 3 4 5 6 7 8 9 10

DEPRESSION / ANXIETY

1 2 3 4 5 6 7 8 9 10

MOOD

☆☆☆☆☆

TODAY'S DIET

WATER INTAKE

BREAKFAST TIME : ....

....

....

....

....

CAL : .... CARBS: .... PROTEIN .... FAT ....

LUNCH TIME : ....

....

....

....

....

CAL : .... CARBS: .... PROTEIN .... FAT ....

DINNER TIME : ....

....

....

....

....

CAL : .... CARBS: .... PROTEIN .... FAT ....

SNACKS TIME: ....

....

....

....

....

CAL : .... CARBS: .... PROTEIN .... FAT ....

REACTION TO FOODS

MEAL : ....

FOOD : ....

SYMPTOMS

....

....

....

....

....

HOW MY APPETITE AFFECTED ?

1 2 3 4 5 6 7 8 9 10

NOT AFFECTED NO APPETITE

HOW IS MY URINATION

1 2 3 4 5 6 7 8 9 10

GOOD WORST

HOW IS MY BOWELS

1 2 3 4 5 6 7 8 9 10

CONSTIPATED LOOSE

EXACERBATING CONDITIONS

CURENT WEATHER

SUNNY OVERCAST

FOGGY

RAINY SNOWY

CURRENT WEATHER AFFECTING ME

1 2 3 4 5 6 7 8 9 10

NONE GREATLY

JOB STRESS LEVEL

1 2 3 4 5 6 7 8 9 10

LOW HIGH

TEMPERATURE

LOW HIGH

FAMILY HOME LIFE STRESS LEVEL

1 2 3 4 5 6 7 8 9 10

LOW HIGH

TOP 3 THINGS I WILL DO TO MY CARE-SELF TODAY

....

....

....

TOP 3 THINGS TO ACCOMPLISH TODAY

....

....

....

TOP 3 HIGHLIGHTS OF MY DAY

....

....

....

NOTES /COMMENTS

....

....

....

....

DATE: .... DAY: ....

DAILY QUOTE

" ....
.... "

	AM	PM
WEIGHT		
TEMPERATURE		
BLOOD PRESSURE		

SUGAR LEVEL

BEFORE BREAKFAST :	AFTER BREAKFAST:
BEFORE LUNCH :	AFTER LUNCH :
BEFORE DINNER :	AFTER DINNER :
BEDTIME :	

SLEEP LAST NIGHT

☐ /HOURS

☐ ☺ ☐ ☹ ☐ 😫

NAPS TODAY

☐ /TOTAL HOURS ☐ /HOW MANY

DRUGS/VITAMINS /HERBS/MEDICATIONS	REASON	DOSAGE	TIME			REACTION

SYMPTOM NOTES

RECURRING SYMPTOMS	
NEW SYMPTOMS	

PAIN SITE IDENTIFICATION

MARK PAINFUL AREAS OF THE BODY

OVERALL MORNING PAIN LEVEL

1 2 3 4 5 6 7 8 9 10

LOW HIGH

OVERALL AFTERNOON PAIN LEVEL

1 2 3 4 5 6 7 8 9 10

LOW HIGH

OVERALL EVENING PAIN LEVEL

1 2 3 4 5 6 7 8 9 10

LOW HIGH

SUSPECTED TRIGGERS

....
....

MEDICATIONS: ....

DID THE MEDICATION HELP? ....

PHYSICAL ACTIVITY

ACTIVITY/ EXERCISE	DURATION	SETS	REPS	CAL	NOTES

FATIGUE

1 2 3 4 5 6 7 8 9 10

DEPRESSION / ANXIETY

1 2 3 4 5 6 7 8 9 10

MOOD

☆ ☆ ☆ ☆ ☆

TODAY'S DIET

WATER INTAKE

BREAKFAST TIME : ....

....

CAL : .... CARBS: .... PROTEIN .... FAT ....

LUNCH TIME : ....

....

CAL : .... CARBS: .... PROTEIN .... FAT ....

DINNER TIME : ....

....

CAL : .... CARBS: .... PROTEIN .... FAT ....

SNACKS TIME: ....

....

CAL : .... CARBS: .... PROTEIN .... FAT ....

REACTION TO FOODS

MEAL : ....

FOOD : ....

SYMPTOMS

....

HOW MY APPETITE AFFECTED ?

1 2 3 4 5 6 7 8 9 10

NOT AFFECTED NO APPETITE

HOW IS MY URINATION

1 2 3 4 5 6 7 8 9 10

GOOD WORST

HOW IS MY BOWELS

1 2 3 4 5 6 7 8 9 10

CONSTIPATED LOOSE

EXACERBATING CONDITIONS

CURENT WEATHER

SUNNY OVERCAST

FOGGY

RAINY SNOWY

CURRENT WEATHER AFFECTING ME

1 2 3 4 5 6 7 8 9 10

NONE GREATLY

JOB STRESS LEVEL

1 2 3 4 5 6 7 8 9 10

LOW HIGH

TEMPERATURE

LOW HIGH

FAMILY HOME LIFE STRESS LEVEL

1 2 3 4 5 6 7 8 9 10

LOW HIGH

TOP 3 THINGS I WILL DO TO MY CARE-SELF TODAY

....

TOP 3 THINGS TO ACCOMPLISH TODAY

....

TOP 3 HIGHLIGHTS OF MY DAY

....

NOTES /COMMENTS

....

DATE: .... DAY: ....

DAILY QUOTE

"
....
....
"

	AM	PM
WEIGHT		
TEMPERATURE		
BLOOD PRESSURE		

SUGAR LEVEL

BEFORE BREAKFAST :	AFTER BREAKFAST:
BEFORE LUNCH :	AFTER LUNCH :
BEFORE DINNER :	AFTER DINNER :

BEDTIME :

SLEEP LAST NIGHT

/HOURS

NAPS TODAY

/TOTAL HOURS /HOW MANY

DRUGS/VITAMINS /HERBS/MEDICATIONS	REASON	DOSAGE	TIME			REACTION

SYMPTOM NOTES

RECURRING SYMPTOMS	
NEW SYMPTOMS	

PAIN SITE IDENTIFICATION

MARK PAINFUL AREAS OF THE BODY

OVERALL MORNING PAIN LEVEL

1 2 3 4 5 6 7 8 9 10

LOW HIGH

OVERALL AFTERNOON PAIN LEVEL

1 2 3 4 5 6 7 8 9 10

LOW HIGH

OVERALL EVENING PAIN LEVEL

1 2 3 4 5 6 7 8 9 10

LOW HIGH

SUSPECTED TRIGGERS

....
....

MEDICATIONS: ....

DID THE MEDICATION HELP? ....

PHYSICAL ACTIVITY

ACTIVITY/ EXERCISE	DURATION	SETS	REPS	CAL	NOTES

FATIGUE

1 2 3 4 5 6 7 8 9 10

DEPRESSION / ANXIETY

1 2 3 4 5 6 7 8 9 10

MOOD

☆☆☆☆☆

TODAY'S DIET

WATER INTAKE

BREAKFAST TIME : ....

CAL : .... CARBS: .... PROTEIN .... FAT ....

LUNCH TIME : ....

CAL : .... CARBS: .... PROTEIN .... FAT ....

DINNER TIME : ....

CAL : .... CARBS: .... PROTEIN .... FAT ....

SNACKS TIME: ....

CAL : .... CARBS: .... PROTEIN .... FAT ....

REACTION TO FOODS

MEAL : ....

FOOD : ....

SYMPTOMS

HOW MY APPETITE AFFECTED ?
1 2 3 4 5 6 7 8 9 10
NOT AFFECTED NO APPETITE

HOW IS MY URINATION
1 2 3 4 5 6 7 8 9 10
GOOD WORST

HOW IS MY BOWELS
1 2 3 4 5 6 7 8 9 10
CONSTIPATED LOOSE

EXACERBATING CONDITIONS

CURENT WEATHER
SUNNY OVERCAST
FOGGY
RAINY SNOWY

CURRENT WEATHER AFFECTING ME
1 2 3 4 5 6 7 8 9 10
NONE GREATLY

JOB STRESS LEVEL
1 2 3 4 5 6 7 8 9 10
LOW HIGH

TEMPERATURE
LOW HIGH

FAMILY HOME LIFE STRESS LEVEL
1 2 3 4 5 6 7 8 9 10
LOW HIGH

TOP 3 THINGS I WILL DO TO MY CARE-SELF TODAY

TOP 3 THINGS TO ACCOMPLISH TODAY

TOP 3 HIGHLIGHTS OF MY DAY

NOTES /COMMENTS

DATE: .... DAY: ....

DAILY QUOTE

"..
...."

	AM	PM
WEIGHT		
TEMPERATURE		
BLOOD PRESSURE		

SUGAR LEVEL

BEFORE BREAKFAST :	AFTER BREAKFAST:
BEFORE LUNCH :	AFTER LUNCH :
BEFORE DINNER :	AFTER DINNER :

BEDTIME :

SLEEP LAST NIGHT

☐ /HOURS

☐ ☺ ☐ ☹ ☐

NAPS TODAY

☐ /TOTAL HOURS ☐ /HOW MANY

DRUGS/VITAMINS /HERBS/MEDICATIONS	REASON	DOSAGE	TIME			REACTION

SYMPTOM NOTES

RECURRING SYMPTOMS	
NEW SYMPTOMS	

PAIN SITE IDENTIFICATION

MARK PAINFUL AREAS OF THE BODY

OVERALL MORNING PAIN LEVEL

1 2 3 4 5 6 7 8 9 10

LOW HIGH

OVERALL AFTERNOON PAIN LEVEL

1 2 3 4 5 6 7 8 9 10

LOW HIGH

OVERALL EVENING PAIN LEVEL

1 2 3 4 5 6 7 8 9 10

LOW HIGH

SUSPECTED TRIGGERS

....
....

MEDICATIONS: ....

DID THE MEDICATION HELP? ....

PHYSICAL ACTIVITY

ACTIVITY/ EXERCISE	DURATION	SETS	REPS	CAL	NOTES

FATIGUE

1 2 3 4 5 6 7 8 9 10

DEPRESSION / ANXIETY

1 2 3 4 5 6 7 8 9 10

MOOD

☆☆☆☆☆

TODAY'S DIET

WATER INTAKE

BREAKFAST TIME : ....

CAL : .... CARBS: .... PROTEIN .... FAT ....

LUNCH TIME : ....

CAL : .... CARBS: .... PROTEIN .... FAT ....

DINNER TIME : ....

CAL : .... CARBS: .... PROTEIN .... FAT ....

SNACKS TIME: ....

CAL : .... CARBS: .... PROTEIN .... FAT ....

REACTION TO FOODS

MEAL : ....

FOOD : ....

SYMPTOMS

HOW MY APPETITE AFFECTED ?

1 2 3 4 5 6 7 8 9 10

NOT AFFECTED NO APPETITE

HOW IS MY URINATION

1 2 3 4 5 6 7 8 9 10

GOOD WORST

HOW IS MY BOWELS

1 2 3 4 5 6 7 8 9 10

CONSTIPATED LOOSE

EXACERBATING CONDITIONS

CURENT WEATHER

SUNNY OVERCAST FOGGY RAINY SNOWY

CURRENT WEATHER AFFECTING ME

1 2 3 4 5 6 7 8 9 10

NONE GREATLY

JOB STRESS LEVEL

1 2 3 4 5 6 7 8 9 10

LOW HIGH

TEMPERATURE

LOW HIGH

FAMILY HOME LIFE STRESS LEVEL

1 2 3 4 5 6 7 8 9 10

LOW HIGH

TOP 3 THINGS I WILL DO TO MY CARE-SELF TODAY

TOP 3 THINGS TO ACCOMPLISH TODAY

TOP 3 HIGHLIGHTS OF MY DAY

NOTES /COMMENTS

DATE: .... DAY: ....

DAILY QUOTE

"..
...."

	AM	PM
WEIGHT		
TEMPERATURE		
BLOOD PRESSURE		

SUGAR LEVEL

BEFORE BREAKFAST :	AFTER BREAKFAST:
BEFORE LUNCH :	AFTER LUNCH :
BEFORE DINNER :	AFTER DINNER :

BEDTIME :

SLEEP LAST NIGHT

☐ /HOURS

☐ ☺ ☐ ☹ ☐

NAPS TODAY

☐ /TOTAL HOURS ☐ /HOW MANY

DRUGS/VITAMINS /HERBS/MEDICATIONS	REASON	DOSAGE	TIME			REACTION

SYMPTOM NOTES

RECURRING SYMPTOMS	
NEW SYMPTOMS	

PAIN SITE IDENTIFICATION

MARK PAINFUL AREAS OF THE BODY

OVERALL MORNING PAIN LEVEL

1 2 3 4 5 6 7 8 9 10

LOW HIGH

OVERALL AFTERNOON PAIN LEVEL

1 2 3 4 5 6 7 8 9 10

LOW HIGH

OVERALL EVENING PAIN LEVEL

1 2 3 4 5 6 7 8 9 10

LOW HIGH

SUSPECTED TRIGGERS

....
....

MEDICATIONS: ....

DID THE MEDICATION HELP? ....

PHYSICAL ACTIVITY

ACTIVITY/ EXERCISE	DURATION	SETS	REPS	CAL	NOTES

FATIGUE

1 2 3 4 5 6 7 8 9 10

DEPRESSION / ANXIETY

1 2 3 4 5 6 7 8 9 10

MOOD

☆☆☆☆☆

TODAY'S DIET

WATER INTAKE

BREAKFAST TIME : ....

....

....

....

....

CAL : .... CARBS: .... PROTEIN .... FAT ....

LUNCH TIME : ....

....

....

....

....

CAL : .... CARBS: .... PROTEIN .... FAT ....

DINNER TIME : ....

....

....

....

....

CAL : .... CARBS: .... PROTEIN .... FAT ....

SNACKS TIME: ....

....

....

....

....

CAL : .... CARBS: .... PROTEIN .... FAT ....

REACTION TO FOODS

MEAL : ....

FOOD : ....

SYMPTOMS

....

....

....

....

....

HOW MY APPETITE AFFECTED ?

1 2 3 4 5 6 7 8 9 10

NOT AFFECTED NO APPETITE

HOW IS MY URINATION

1 2 3 4 5 6 7 8 9 10

GOOD WORST

HOW IS MY BOWELS

1 2 3 4 5 6 7 8 9 10

CONSTIPATED LOOSE

EXACERBATING CONDITIONS

CURENT WEATHER

SUNNY OVERCAST

FOGGY

RAINY SNOWY

CURRENT WEATHER AFFECTING ME

1 2 3 4 5 6 7 8 9 10

NONE GREATLY

JOB STRESS LEVEL

1 2 3 4 5 6 7 8 9 10

LOW HIGH

TEMPERATURE

LOW HIGH

FAMILY HOME LIFE STRESS LEVEL

1 2 3 4 5 6 7 8 9 10

LOW HIGH

TOP 3 THINGS I WILL DO TO MY CARE-SELF TODAY

....

....

....

TOP 3 THINGS TO ACCOMPLISH TODAY

....

....

....

TOP 3 HIGHLIGHTS OF MY DAY

....

....

....

NOTES /COMMENTS

....

....

....

....

DATE: .... DAY: ....

DAILY QUOTE

" ....
.... "

	AM	PM
WEIGHT		
TEMPERATURE		
BLOOD PRESSURE		

SUGAR LEVEL

BEFORE BREAKFAST :	AFTER BREAKFAST:
BEFORE LUNCH :	AFTER LUNCH :
BEFORE DINNER :	AFTER DINNER :

BEDTIME :

SLEEP LAST NIGHT

☐ /HOURS

☐ ☺ ☐ ☹ ☐ 😫

NAPS TODAY

☐ /TOTAL HOURS ☐ /HOW MANY

DRUGS/VITAMINS /HERBS/MEDICATIONS	REASON	DOSAGE	TIME			REACTION

SYMPTOM NOTES

RECURRING SYMPTOMS	
NEW SYMPTOMS	

PAIN SITE IDENTIFICATION

MARK PAINFUL AREAS OF THE BODY

OVERALL MORNING PAIN LEVEL

1 2 3 4 5 6 7 8 9 10

LOW HIGH

OVERALL EVENING PAIN LEVEL

1 2 3 4 5 6 7 8 9 10

LOW HIGH

OVERALL AFTERNOON PAIN LEVEL

1 2 3 4 5 6 7 8 9 10

LOW HIGH

SUSPECTED TRIGGERS

....
....

MEDICATIONS: ....

DID THE MEDICATION HELP? ....

PHYSICAL ACTIVITY

ACTIVITY/ EXERCISE	DURATION	SETS	REPS	CAL	NOTES

FATIGUE

1 2 3 4 5 6 7 8 9 10

DEPRESSION / ANXIETY

1 2 3 4 5 6 7 8 9 10

MOOD

☆ ☆ ☆ ☆ ☆

TODAY'S DIET

WATER INTAKE

BREAKFAST TIME : ....

CAL : .... CARBS: .... PROTEIN .... FAT ....

LUNCH TIME : ....

CAL : .... CARBS: .... PROTEIN .... FAT ....

DINNER TIME : ....

CAL : .... CARBS: .... PROTEIN .... FAT ....

SNACKS TIME: ....

CAL : .... CARBS: .... PROTEIN .... FAT ....

REACTION TO FOODS

MEAL : ....

FOOD : ....

SYMPTOMS

HOW MY APPETITE AFFECTED ?

1 2 3 4 5 6 7 8 9 10

NOT AFFECTED NO APPETITE

HOW IS MY URINATION

1 2 3 4 5 6 7 8 9 10

GOOD WORST

HOW IS MY BOWELS

1 2 3 4 5 6 7 8 9 10

CONSTIPATED LOOSE

EXACERBATING CONDITIONS

CURENT WEATHER

SUNNY OVERCAST

FOGGY

RAINY SNOWY

CURRENT WEATHER AFFECTING ME

1 2 3 4 5 6 7 8 9 10

NONE GREATLY

JOB STRESS LEVEL

1 2 3 4 5 6 7 8 9 10

LOW HIGH

TEMPERATURE

LOW HIGH

FAMILY HOME LIFE STRESS LEVEL

1 2 3 4 5 6 7 8 9 10

LOW HIGH

TOP 3 THINGS I WILL DO TO MY CARE-SELF TODAY

TOP 3 THINGS TO ACCOMPLISH TODAY

TOP 3 HIGHLIGHTS OF MY DAY

NOTES /COMMENTS

DATE: .... DAY: ....

DAILY QUOTE

"..
...."

	AM	PM
WEIGHT		
TEMPERATURE		
BLOOD PRESSURE		

SUGAR LEVEL

BEFORE BREAKFAST :	AFTER BREAKFAST:
BEFORE LUNCH :	AFTER LUNCH :
BEFORE DINNER :	AFTER DINNER :

BEDTIME :

SLEEP LAST NIGHT

☐ /HOURS

☐ ☺ ☐ ☹ ☐

NAPS TODAY

☐ /TOTAL HOURS ☐ /HOW MANY

DRUGS/VITAMINS /HERBS/MEDICATIONS	REASON	DOSAGE	TIME			REACTION

SYMPTOM NOTES

RECURRING SYMPTOMS	
NEW SYMPTOMS	

PAIN SITE IDENTIFICATION

MARK PAINFUL AREAS OF THE BODY

OVERALL MORNING PAIN LEVEL

1 2 3 4 5 6 7 8 9 10

LOW HIGH

OVERALL AFTERNOON PAIN LEVEL

1 2 3 4 5 6 7 8 9 10

LOW HIGH

OVERALL EVENING PAIN LEVEL

1 2 3 4 5 6 7 8 9 10

LOW HIGH

SUSPECTED TRIGGERS

....
....

MEDICATIONS: ....

DID THE MEDICATION HELP? ....

PHYSICAL ACTIVITY

ACTIVITY/ EXERCISE	DURATION	SETS	REPS	CAL	NOTES

FATIGUE

1 2 3 4 5 6 7 8 9 10

DEPRESSION / ANXIETY

1 2 3 4 5 6 7 8 9 10

MOOD

☆☆☆☆☆

TODAY'S DIET

WATER INTAKE

BREAKFAST
TIME : ....
CAL : .... CARBS: .... PROTEIN .... FAT ....

LUNCH
TIME : ....
CAL : .... CARBS: .... PROTEIN .... FAT ....

DINNER
TIME : ....
CAL : .... CARBS: .... PROTEIN .... FAT ....

SNACKS
TIME: ....
CAL : .... CARBS: .... PROTEIN .... FAT ....

REACTION TO FOODS
MEAL : ....
FOOD : ....

SYMPTOMS

HOW MY APPETITE AFFECTED ?
1 2 3 4 5 6 7 8 9 10
NOT AFFECTED NO APPETITE

HOW IS MY URINATION
1 2 3 4 5 6 7 8 9 10
GOOD WORST

HOW IS MY BOWELS
1 2 3 4 5 6 7 8 9 10
CONSTIPATED LOOSE

EXACERBATING CONDITIONS

CURENT WEATHER
SUNNY OVERCAST
FOGGY
RAINY SNOWY

CURRENT WEATHER AFFECTING ME
1 2 3 4 5 6 7 8 9 10
NONE GREATLY

JOB STRESS LEVEL
1 2 3 4 5 6 7 8 9 10
LOW HIGH

TEMPERATURE
LOW HIGH

FAMILY HOME LIFE STRESS LEVEL
1 2 3 4 5 6 7 8 9 10
LOW HIGH

TOP 3 THINGS I WILL DO TO MY CARE-SELF TODAY

TOP 3 THINGS TO ACCOMPLISH TODAY

TOP 3 HIGHLIGHTS OF MY DAY

NOTES /COMMENTS

DATE: .... DAY: ....

DAILY QUOTE

" ....
.... "

	AM	PM
WEIGHT		
TEMPERATURE		
BLOOD PRESSURE		

SUGAR LEVEL

BEFORE BREAKFAST :	AFTER BREAKFAST:
BEFORE LUNCH :	AFTER LUNCH :
BEFORE DINNER :	AFTER DINNER :

BEDTIME :

SLEEP LAST NIGHT

☐ /HOURS

☐ ☺ ☐ ☹ ☐

NAPS TODAY

☐ /TOTAL HOURS ☐ /HOW MANY

DRUGS/VITAMINS /HERBS/MEDICATIONS	REASON	DOSAGE	TIME			REACTION

SYMPTOM NOTES

RECURRING SYMPTOMS	
NEW SYMPTOMS	

PAIN SITE IDENTIFICATION

MARK PAINFUL AREAS OF THE BODY

OVERALL MORNING PAIN LEVEL

1 2 3 4 5 6 7 8 9 10

LOW HIGH

OVERALL AFTERNOON PAIN LEVEL

1 2 3 4 5 6 7 8 9 10

LOW HIGH

OVERALL EVENING PAIN LEVEL

1 2 3 4 5 6 7 8 9 10

LOW HIGH

SUSPECTED TRIGGERS

....
....

MEDICATIONS: ....

DID THE MEDICATION HELP? ....

PHYSICAL ACTIVITY

ACTIVITY/ EXERCISE	DURATION	SETS	REPS	CAL	NOTES

FATIGUE

1 2 3 4 5 6 7 8 9 10

DEPRESSION / ANXIETY

1 2 3 4 5 6 7 8 9 10

MOOD

☆☆☆☆☆

TODAY'S DIET

WATER INTAKE

BREAKFAST TIME : ....

....
....
....
....

CAL : .... CARBS: .... PROTEIN .... FAT ....

LUNCH TIME : ....

....
....
....
....

CAL : .... CARBS: .... PROTEIN .... FAT ....

DINNER TIME : ....

....
....
....
....

CAL : .... CARBS: .... PROTEIN .... FAT ....

SNACKS TIME: ....

....
....
....
....

CAL : .... CARBS: .... PROTEIN .... FAT ....

REACTION TO FOODS

MEAL : ....

FOOD : ....

SYMPTOMS

....
....
....
....
....

HOW MY APPETITE AFFECTED ?

1 2 3 4 5 6 7 8 9 10

NOT AFFECTED NO APPETITE

HOW IS MY URINATION

1 2 3 4 5 6 7 8 9 10

GOOD WORST

HOW IS MY BOWELS

1 2 3 4 5 6 7 8 9 10

CONSTIPATED LOOSE

EXACERBATING CONDITIONS

CURENT WEATHER

SUNNY OVERCAST

FOGGY

RAINY SNOWY

CURRENT WEATHER AFFECTING ME

1 2 3 4 5 6 7 8 9 10

NONE GREATLY

JOB STRESS LEVEL

1 2 3 4 5 6 7 8 9 10

LOW HIGH

TEMPERATURE

LOW HIGH

FAMILY HOME LIFE STRESS LEVEL

1 2 3 4 5 6 7 8 9 10

LOW HIGH

TOP 3 THINGS I WILL DO TO MY CARE-SELF TODAY

....
....
....

TOP 3 THINGS TO ACCOMPLISH TODAY

....
....
....

TOP 3 HIGHLIGHTS OF MY DAY

....
....
....

NOTES /COMMENTS

....
....
....
....

DATE: .... **DAY:** ....

DAILY QUOTE

"..
...."

	AM	PM
WEIGHT		
TEMPERATURE		
BLOOD PRESSURE		

SUGAR LEVEL

BEFORE BREAKFAST :	AFTER BREAKFAST:
BEFORE LUNCH :	AFTER LUNCH :
BEFORE DINNER :	AFTER DINNER :

BEDTIME :

SLEEP LAST NIGHT

☐ /HOURS

☐ ☺ ☐ ☹ ☐

NAPS TODAY

☐ /TOTAL HOURS ☐ /HOW MANY

DRUGS/VITAMINS /HERBS/MEDICATIONS	REASON	DOSAGE	TIME			REACTION

SYMPTOM NOTES

RECURRING SYMPTOMS	
NEW SYMPTOMS	

PAIN SITE IDENTIFICATION

MARK PAINFUL AREAS OF THE BODY

OVERALL MORNING PAIN LEVEL

1 2 3 4 5 6 7 8 9 10

LOW HIGH

OVERALL AFTERNOON PAIN LEVEL

1 2 3 4 5 6 7 8 9 10

LOW HIGH

OVERALL EVENING PAIN LEVEL

1 2 3 4 5 6 7 8 9 10

LOW HIGH

SUSPECTED TRIGGERS

....
....

MEDICATIONS: ....

DID THE MEDICATION HELP? ....

PHYSICAL ACTIVITY

ACTIVITY/ EXERCISE	DURATION	SETS	REPS	CAL	NOTES

FATIGUE

1 2 3 4 5 6 7 8 9 10

DEPRESSION / ANXIETY

1 2 3 4 5 6 7 8 9 10

MOOD

☆☆☆☆☆

TODAY'S DIET

WATER INTAKE

BREAKFAST TIME : ....

CAL : .... CARBS: .... PROTEIN .... FAT ....

LUNCH TIME : ....

CAL : .... CARBS: .... PROTEIN .... FAT ....

DINNER TIME : ....

CAL : .... CARBS: .... PROTEIN .... FAT ....

SNACKS TIME: ....

CAL : .... CARBS: .... PROTEIN .... FAT ....

REACTION TO FOODS

MEAL : ....

FOOD : ....

SYMPTOMS

HOW MY APPETITE AFFECTED ?

1 2 3 4 5 6 7 8 9 10

NOT AFFECTED NO APPETITE

HOW IS MY URINATION

1 2 3 4 5 6 7 8 9 10

GOOD WORST

HOW IS MY BOWELS

1 2 3 4 5 6 7 8 9 10

CONSTIPATED LOOSE

EXACERBATING CONDITIONS

CURENT WEATHER

SUNNY OVERCAST

FOGGY

RAINY SNOWY

CURRENT WEATHER AFFECTING ME

1 2 3 4 5 6 7 8 9 10

NONE GREATLY

JOB STRESS LEVEL

1 2 3 4 5 6 7 8 9 10

LOW HIGH

TEMPERATURE

LOW HIGH

FAMILY HOME LIFE STRESS LEVEL

1 2 3 4 5 6 7 8 9 10

LOW HIGH

TOP 3 THINGS I WILL DO TO MY CARE-SELF TODAY

TOP 3 THINGS TO ACCOMPLISH TODAY

TOP 3 HIGHLIGHTS OF MY DAY

NOTES /COMMENTS

DATE: .... DAY: ....

DAILY QUOTE

" ....
.... "

	AM	PM
WEIGHT		
TEMPERATURE		
BLOOD PRESSURE		

SUGAR LEVEL

BEFORE BREAKFAST :	AFTER BREAKFAST:
BEFORE LUNCH :	AFTER LUNCH :
BEFORE DINNER :	AFTER DINNER :

BEDTIME :

SLEEP LAST NIGHT

☐ /HOURS

☐ ☺ ☐ ☹ ☐

NAPS TODAY

☐ /TOTAL HOURS ☐ /HOW MANY

DRUGS/VITAMINS /HERBS/MEDICATIONS	REASON	DOSAGE	TIME			REACTION

SYMPTOM NOTES

RECURRING SYMPTOMS	
NEW SYMPTOMS	

PAIN SITE IDENTIFICATION

MARK PAINFUL AREAS OF THE BODY

OVERALL MORNING PAIN LEVEL

1 2 3 4 5 6 7 8 9 10

LOW HIGH

OVERALL AFTERNOON PAIN LEVEL

1 2 3 4 5 6 7 8 9 10

LOW HIGH

OVERALL EVENING PAIN LEVEL

1 2 3 4 5 6 7 8 9 10

LOW HIGH

SUSPECTED TRIGGERS

....
....

MEDICATIONS: ....

DID THE MEDICATION HELP? ....

PHYSICAL ACTIVITY

ACTIVITY/ EXERCISE	DURATION	SETS	REPS	CAL	NOTES

FATIGUE

1 2 3 4 5 6 7 8 9 10

DEPRESSION / ANXIETY

1 2 3 4 5 6 7 8 9 10

MOOD

☆☆☆☆☆

TODAY'S DIET

WATER INTAKE

BREAKFAST TIME : ....

CAL : .... CARBS: .... PROTEIN .... FAT ....

LUNCH TIME : ....

CAL : .... CARBS: .... PROTEIN .... FAT ....

DINNER TIME : ....

CAL : .... CARBS: .... PROTEIN .... FAT ....

SNACKS TIME: ....

CAL : .... CARBS: .... PROTEIN .... FAT ....

REACTION TO FOODS

MEAL : ....

FOOD : ....

SYMPTOMS

HOW MY APPETITE AFFECTED ?

1 2 3 4 5 6 7 8 9 10

NOT AFFECTED NO APPETITE

HOW IS MY URINATION

1 2 3 4 5 6 7 8 9 10

GOOD WORST

HOW IS MY BOWELS

1 2 3 4 5 6 7 8 9 10

CONSTIPATED LOOSE

EXACERBATING CONDITIONS

CURENT WEATHER

SUNNY OVERCAST

FOGGY

RAINY SNOWY

CURRENT WEATHER AFFECTING ME

1 2 3 4 5 6 7 8 9 10

NONE GREATLY

JOB STRESS LEVEL

1 2 3 4 5 6 7 8 9 10

LOW HIGH

TEMPERATURE

LOW HIGH

FAMILY HOME LIFE STRESS LEVEL

1 2 3 4 5 6 7 8 9 10

LOW HIGH

TOP 3 THINGS I WILL DO TO MY CARE-SELF TODAY

TOP 3 THINGS TO ACCOMPLISH TODAY

TOP 3 HIGHLIGHTS OF MY DAY

NOTES /COMMENTS

DATE: .... DAY: ....

DAILY QUOTE

"..
...."

	AM	PM
WEIGHT		
TEMPERATURE		
BLOOD PRESSURE		

SUGAR LEVEL

BEFORE BREAKFAST :	AFTER BREAKFAST:
BEFORE LUNCH :	AFTER LUNCH :
BEFORE DINNER :	AFTER DINNER :

BEDTIME :

SLEEP LAST NIGHT

/HOURS

NAPS TODAY

/TOTAL HOURS /HOW MANY

DRUGS/VITAMINS /HERBS/MEDICATIONS	REASON	DOSAGE	TIME			REACTION

SYMPTOM NOTES

RECURRING SYMPTOMS	
NEW SYMPTOMS	

PAIN SITE IDENTIFICATION

MARK PAINFUL AREAS OF THE BODY

OVERALL MORNING PAIN LEVEL

1 2 3 4 5 6 7 8 9 10

LOW HIGH

OVERALL AFTERNOON PAIN LEVEL

1 2 3 4 5 6 7 8 9 10

LOW HIGH

OVERALL EVENING PAIN LEVEL

1 2 3 4 5 6 7 8 9 10

LOW HIGH

SUSPECTED TRIGGERS

....
....

MEDICATIONS: ....

DID THE MEDICATION HELP? ....

PHYSICAL ACTIVITY

ACTIVITY/ EXERCISE	DURATION	SETS	REPS	CAL	NOTES

FATIGUE

1 2 3 4 5 6 7 8 9 10

DEPRESSION / ANXIETY

1 2 3 4 5 6 7 8 9 10

MOOD

☆☆☆☆☆

TODAY'S DIET

WATER INTAKE

BREAKFAST TIME : ....

CAL : .... CARBS: .... PROTEIN .... FAT ....

LUNCH TIME : ....

CAL : .... CARBS: .... PROTEIN .... FAT ....

DINNER TIME : ....

CAL : .... CARBS: .... PROTEIN .... FAT ....

SNACKS TIME: ....

CAL : .... CARBS: .... PROTEIN .... FAT ....

REACTION TO FOODS

MEAL : ....

FOOD : ....

SYMPTOMS

....

HOW MY APPETITE AFFECTED ?

1 2 3 4 5 6 7 8 9 10

NOT AFFECTED NO APPETITE

HOW IS MY URINATION

1 2 3 4 5 6 7 8 9 10

GOOD WORST

HOW IS MY BOWELS

1 2 3 4 5 6 7 8 9 10

CONSTIPATED LOOSE

EXACERBATING CONDITIONS

CURENT WEATHER

SUNNY OVERCAST

FOGGY

RAINY SNOWY

CURRENT WEATHER AFFECTING ME

1 2 3 4 5 6 7 8 9 10

NONE GREATLY

JOB STRESS LEVEL

1 2 3 4 5 6 7 8 9 10

LOW HIGH

TEMPERATURE

LOW HIGH

FAMILY HOME LIFE STRESS LEVEL

1 2 3 4 5 6 7 8 9 10

LOW HIGH

TOP 3 THINGS I WILL DO TO MY CARE-SELF TODAY

....

TOP 3 THINGS TO ACCOMPLISH TODAY

....

TOP 3 HIGHLIGHTS OF MY DAY

....

NOTES /COMMENTS

....

DATE: .... DAY: ....

DAILY QUOTE

" ....
.... "

	AM	PM
WEIGHT		
TEMPERATURE		
BLOOD PRESSURE		

SUGAR LEVEL

BEFORE BREAKFAST :	AFTER BREAKFAST:
BEFORE LUNCH :	AFTER LUNCH :
BEFORE DINNER :	AFTER DINNER :
BEDTIME :	

SLEEP LAST NIGHT

☐ /HOURS

☐ ☺ ☐ ☹ ☐ 😫

NAPS TODAY

☐ /TOTAL HOURS ☐ /HOW MANY

DRUGS/VITAMINS /HERBS/MEDICATIONS	REASON	DOSAGE	TIME			REACTION

SYMPTOM NOTES

RECURRING SYMPTOMS	
NEW SYMPTOMS	

PAIN SITE IDENTIFICATION

MARK PAINFUL AREAS OF THE BODY

OVERALL MORNING PAIN LEVEL

1 2 3 4 5 6 7 8 9 10

LOW HIGH

OVERALL AFTERNOON PAIN LEVEL

1 2 3 4 5 6 7 8 9 10

LOW HIGH

OVERALL EVENING PAIN LEVEL

1 2 3 4 5 6 7 8 9 10

LOW HIGH

SUSPECTED TRIGGERS

....
....

MEDICATIONS: ....

DID THE MEDICATION HELP? ....

PHYSICAL ACTIVITY

ACTIVITY/ EXERCISE	DURATION	SETS	REPS	CAL	NOTES

FATIGUE

1 2 3 4 5 6 7 8 9 10

DEPRESSION / ANXIETY

1 2 3 4 5 6 7 8 9 10

MOOD

☆ ☆ ☆ ☆ ☆

TODAY'S DIET

WATER INTAKE

BREAKFAST TIME : ....

CAL : .... CARBS: .... PROTEIN .... FAT ....

LUNCH TIME : ....

CAL : .... CARBS: .... PROTEIN .... FAT ....

DINNER TIME : ....

CAL : .... CARBS: .... PROTEIN .... FAT ....

SNACKS TIME: ....

CAL : .... CARBS: .... PROTEIN .... FAT ....

REACTION TO FOODS

MEAL : ....

FOOD : ....

SYMPTOMS

HOW MY APPETITE AFFECTED ?
1 2 3 4 5 6 7 8 9 10
NOT AFFECTED NO APPETITE

HOW IS MY URINATION
1 2 3 4 5 6 7 8 9 10
GOOD WORST

HOW IS MY BOWELS
1 2 3 4 5 6 7 8 9 10
CONSTIPATED LOOSE

EXACERBATING CONDITIONS

CURENT WEATHER
SUNNY OVERCAST
FOGGY
RAINY SNOWY

CURRENT WEATHER AFFECTING ME
1 2 3 4 5 6 7 8 9 10
NONE GREATLY

JOB STRESS LEVEL
1 2 3 4 5 6 7 8 9 10
LOW HIGH

TEMPERATURE
LOW HIGH

FAMILY HOME LIFE STRESS LEVEL
1 2 3 4 5 6 7 8 9 10
LOW HIGH

TOP 3 THINGS I WILL DO TO MY CARE-SELF TODAY

TOP 3 THINGS TO ACCOMPLISH TODAY

TOP 3 HIGHLIGHTS OF MY DAY

NOTES /COMMENTS

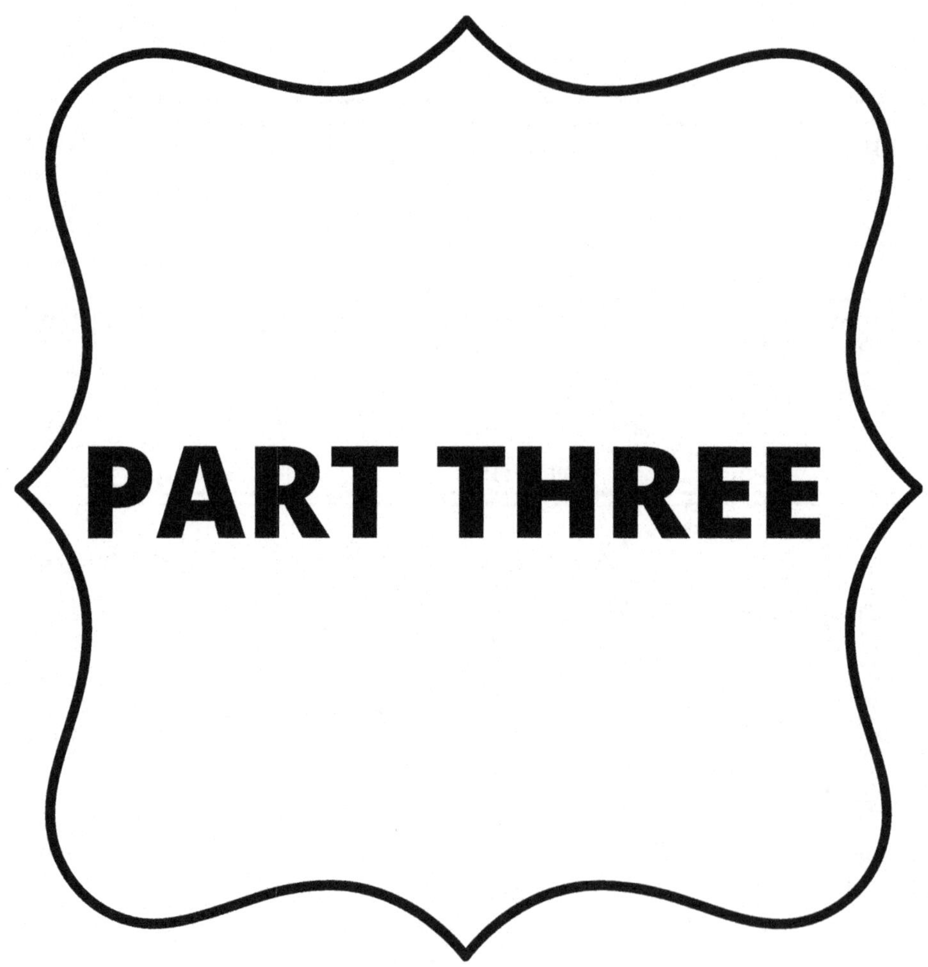

PART THREE

Health Screening

SCREENING TEST	DATE COMPLETED					
ROUTINE PHYSICAL						
BODY MASS INDEX						
CHOLESTEROL						
BLOOD PRESSURE						
HEPATITIS B						
STDS						
HEMOGLOBIN A1C (DIABETES)						
COLORECTAL CANCER SCREEN						
SKIN CANCER SCREEN						
HEARING EXAM						
VISION EXAM						
DENTAL EXAM						
IMMUNIZATIONS						
TETANUS						
INFLUENZA VACCINE						
PNEUMOCOCCAL						
HEPATITIS B						
ZOSTER (SHINGLES)						
WOMEN						
PAP/CHLAMYDIA						
CLINICAL BREAST EXAM						
MAMMOGRAM						
BONE DENSITY						

Appointments

SPECIALIST DETAILS	REASON	DATE	TIME	FOLLOW UP APP.

Medical Check Up Log

NAME : DOCTOR:

Date ____________ Next appt ____________

Descriptions : NOTES :

NAME : DOCTOR:

Date ____________ Next appt ____________

Descriptions : NOTES :

NAME : DOCTOR:

Date ____________ Next appt ____________

Descriptions : NOTES :

NAME : DOCTOR:

Date ____________ Next appt ____________

Descriptions : NOTES :

NAME : DOCTOR:

Date ____________ Next appt ____________

Descriptions : NOTES :

Medical Check Up Log

NAME : DOCTOR:

Date ____________ Next appt ____________

Descriptions : NOTES :

NAME : DOCTOR:

Date ____________ Next appt ____________

Descriptions : NOTES :

NAME : DOCTOR:

Date ____________ Next appt ____________

Descriptions : NOTES :

NAME : DOCTOR:

Date ____________ Next appt ____________

Descriptions : NOTES :

NAME : DOCTOR:

Date ____________ Next appt ____________

Descriptions : NOTES :

Dental Chek Up

NAME : **DENTIST:**

Date ____________ **Next appt** ____________

Descriptions :

NOTES :

NAME : **DENTIST:**

Date ____________ **Next appt** ____________

Descriptions :

NOTES :

NAME : **DENTIST:**

Date ____________ **Next appt** ____________

Descriptions :

NOTES :

NAME : **DENTIST:**

Date ____________ **Next appt** ____________

Descriptions :

NOTES :

NAME : **DENTIST:**

Date ____________ **Next appt** ____________

Descriptions :

NOTES :

Medical Tests

Date	Test Type	Details	Result Notes

Medical Contact List

NAME: **SPECIALITY:**

Phone N°: ______________ **Address :** ______________

Email: ______________ ______________

Notes :

NAME: **SPECIALITY:**

Phone N°: ______________ **Address :** ______________

Email: ______________ ______________

Notes :

NAME: **SPECIALITY:**

Phone N°: ______________ **Address :** ______________

Email: ______________ ______________

Notes :

NAME: **SPECIALITY:**

Phone N°: ______________ **Address :** ______________

Email: ______________ ______________

Notes :

Medical Contact List

NAME: SPECIALITY:

Phone N°: Address :

Email:

Notes :

NAME: SPECIALITY:

Phone N°: Address :

Email:

Notes :

NAME: SPECIALITY:

Phone N°: Address :

Email:

Notes :

NAME: SPECIALITY:

Phone N°: Address :

Email:

Notes :

Insurance Contact List

COMPANY: **POLICY NUMBER:**

Insurance type ____________ Address ____________

Contact ____________ ____________

Email ____________ Website ____________

Notes :

COMPANY: **POLICY NUMBER:**

Insurance type ____________ Address ____________

Contact ____________ ____________

Email ____________ Website ____________

Notes :

COMPANY: **POLICY NUMBER:**

Insurance type ____________ Address ____________

Contact ____________ ____________

Email ____________ Website ____________

Notes :

COMPANY: **POLICY NUMBER:**

Insurance type ____________ Address ____________

Contact ____________ ____________

Email ____________ Website ____________

Notes :

Medical expenses

DATE	EXPENSE DETAILS	COST	AMOUNT PAID	AMOUNT OWING

QUESTIONS / NOTES

B¹ - 1.

B¹ Deficiency

Building Myelin Energy Production Muscle Coordination

1. Nerve Pain (Hands & Feet) Your body uses B¹ (thiamine) to build and protect the coating around your nerves called myelin.

Nerve Pain - this usually happens to people with high blood sugars or diabetics.

2. Anxiety & Stress

3.

QUESTIONS / NOTES

QUESTIONS / NOTES

Made in United States
North Haven, CT
17 March 2022